"In the Daoist tradition, cultivatio Eight Extraordinary Meridians prov enlightenment or immortality. Th QuanZhenNanZong 全真南宗 (the Southern Complete Reality School), Zhang Ziyang 張紫陽, stated that those who are able to open the Eight Extraordinary Meridians will obtain the Dao. I recommend David Twicken's *Eight Extraordinary Channels* to Chinese medicine and qi gong practitioners interested in working with the physical and spiritual layers through these extraordinary meridians."

—*Master Zhongxian Wu, lifelong Daoist practitioner and author of eleven books on Chinese wisdom traditions*

"*Eight Extraordinary Channels* is an insightful and eminently practical presentation of the core meridians in the human body that hold most of life's potential. It covers the Eight Channels in theory, clinical application, and Daoist self-cultivation. Clear and systematic, the book is a potent resource for anyone involved in Chinese medicine."

—*Livia Kohn, Ph.D., Professor Emerita of Religion and East Asian Studies, Boston University*

"Close to turning of the Dao, the Eight Extraordinary Channels correlate to eight directions of space. David Twicken's clear introduction to these channels and their Nei Dan applications allows the reader a direct alchemical and meditative experience. Such a view is essential to best practices in qi gong, herbs and acupuncture. A great contribution!"

—*William Morris, Ph.D., author of* Li Shi Zhen Pulse Studies: An Illustrated Guide

"Twicken illuminates the missing link between Chinese medicine and Taoist spiritual practice, making it essential reading for both healers and adepts. His book is far superior to existing Eight Extra Vessel literature with its wealth of historical detail and rare clinical protocols that penetrate deep ancestral and constitutional issues. In my 35 years' experience, any healer who opens their Eight Extra Channels will quickly improve their clinical success rate. More important, they will open wide the 'Eight Big Rivers' of prenatal Jing. Also known as 'Eight Psychic Channels', in Taoist internal alchemy they are linked together to open the Microcosmic Orbit—the key to whole body enlightenment and long life."

—*Michael Winn, founder www.HealingTaoUSA.com and co-writer with Mantak Chia of seven books on Nei Dan Gong*

EIGHT EXTRAORDINARY CHANNELS

Qi Jing Ba Mai

by the same author

I Ching Acupuncture—The Balance Method
Clinical Applications of the Ba Gua and I Ching
ISBN 978 1 84819 074 0
eISBN 978 0 85701 064 3

of related interest

Daoist Nei Gong
The Philosophical Art of Change
Damo Mitchell
Foreword by Dr Cindy Engel
ISBN 978 1 84819 065 8
eISBN 978 0 85701 033 9

Heavenly Streams
Meridian Theory in Nei Gong
Damo Mitchell
Foreword by Robert Aspell
ISBN 978 1 84819 116 7
eISBN 978 0 85701 101 5

The Great Intent
Acupuncture Odes, Songs and Rhymes
Richard Bertschinger
ISBN 978 1 84819 132 7
eISBN 978 0 85701 111 4

Heavenly Stems and Earthly Branches—TianGan DiZhi
The Keys to the Sublime
Master Zhongxian Wu and Dr Karin Taylor Wu
ISBN 978 1 84819 151 8
Card Set ISBN 978 1 84819 150 1

EIGHT EXTRAORDINARY CHANNELS

QI JING BA MAI

A HANDBOOK FOR CLINICAL
PRACTICE AND NEI DAN
INNER MEDITATION

DR. DAVID TWICKEN DOM, L.AC.

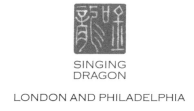

SINGING
DRAGON

LONDON AND PHILADELPHIA

Figures 5.1, 6.1, 7.1, 9.1, 10.1, 12.1, 13.1, 14.1, 21.2, 22.1, 22.2
reproduced with kind permission from Dr. Jerry Alan Johnson.
Figures 20.2, 21.1, 21.3, 23.1, 24.1, 26.2 reproduced with kind permission from Mantak Chia.

First published in 2013
by Singing Dragon
an imprint of Jessica Kingsley Publishers
116 Pentonville Road
London N1 9JB, UK
and
400 Market Street, Suite 400
Philadelphia, PA 19106, USA

www.singingdragon.com

Library of Congress Cataloging in Publication Data
Twicken, David.
   Eight extraordinary channels : qi jing ba mai : a handbook for clinical practice and nei dan inner
meditation / Dr. David Twicken DOM, LAC.
      pages cm
   Includes bibliographical references and index.
   ISBN 978-1-84819-148-8 (alk. paper)
  1. Acupuncture points. 2. Medicine, Chinese--Philosophy.
 3. Meditation. I. Title. II. Title: Qi jing ba
mai.
   RM184.5.T95 2013
   615.8'222--dc23
                              2013012243

British Library Cataloguing in Publication Data
A CIP catalogue record for this book is available from the British Library

ISBN 978 1 84819 148 8
eISBN 978 0 85701 137 4

Printed and bound in Great Britain

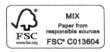

CONTENTS

PART I THE EIGHT EXTRAORDINARY CHANNELS IN CLINICAL PRACTICE

PART II THE EIGHT EXTRAORDINARY CHANNELS IN NEI DAN MEDITATION

DISCLAIMER

The information in this book is based on the author's knowledge and personal experience. It is presented for educational purposes to assist the reader in expanding his or her knowledge of Chinese philosophy and medicine. The techniques and practices are to be used at the reader's own discretion and liability. The author is not responsible in any manner whatsoever for any physical injury that may occur as a result of following instructions in this book.

Acknowledgments

I have been fortunate to study with some very special people. One common quality among all of them was their encouragement to study a wide range of teachings. I would like to give special thanks to Master Mary Chow, who taught me how to bring joy and love to practicing Tai Chi Chuan; to Master Joseph Yu for sharing the importance of studying classics and learning to apply them in practice; and to Master Peter Leung for showing how to bring creativity into the practice of Chinese metaphysics. A special thank you goes to Master Mantak Chia for sharing qi gong, meditation, internal alchemy, and Taoism with compassion, respect, and love, and to Master Jeffrey Yuen for sharing his Taoist tradition in a humble, caring, and inspirational way.

I would like to thank Jessica Kingsley, and the team at Singing Dragon, for publishing this book. Thank you, Molly Maguire, my very good friend Gregory E. Leblanc, L.Ac., and Douglas Eisentark, L.Ac., for your editorial contributions. And thank you, Steven Sy, for your editing contribution on the Nei Dan chapters (Chapters 20–26).

Credits

Dr. Jerry Alan Johnson, Chinese Medical Qi Gong Therapy, International Institute of Medical Qi Gong:
Figure 5.1 The Chong channel
Figure 6.1 The Ren channel
Figure 7.1 The Du channel
Figure 9.1 The Yang Wei channel
Figure 10.1 The Yin Wei channel
Figure 12.1 The Yang Qiao channel
Figure 13.1 The Yin Qiao channel
Figure 14.1 The Dai channel
Figure 21.2 The lower Dan Tian

PREFACE

The Eight Extraordinary Channels are one of the most interesting and clinically important aspects of Chinese medicine, qi gong, and Nei Dan. This book introduces theory and clinical applications of the Eight Extraordinary Channels. The information in this book is based on my experiences studying, practicing, and teaching Chinese medicine and the Taoist arts, including acupuncture, herbal medicine, qi gong, Nei Dan, I Ching, feng shui, Qi Men Dun Jia, and Chinese astrology.

Most of the books on the Eight Extraordinary Channels are textbooks designed for Chinese medical schools. The material in those books includes a basic understanding of the channels. There are a few books that are translations of past works. Both provide contributions to understanding these channels. My intention in writing this book is to present ways of understanding these channels that are not commonly available. My goal was to write a book focused on clinical practice, with an emphasis on the psycho-emotional, spiritual, alchemical, and inner meditative aspects of the Eight Extraordinary Channels. Treatment strategies, methods, and cases are presented, providing a variety of clinical approaches. Please be creative and flexible in creating clinical applications. The material in this book is designed to provide the foundation knowledge to customize treatments for each person. The key to creating individual treatment plans is having a wide understanding of channel theory, pathways, and the points on the channels.

The ancient Chinese had a unique insight about the relationship between nature and humanity. This relationship is expressed in the ancient diagram: the Nei Jing Tu. This diagram reveals the process of transforming Jing to qi to *shen*. The Eight Extraordinary Channels play a major role in that transformation process. A unique inner meditation called Nei Dan (Inner Pill) is presented in Chapters 20–26. This Nei Dan allows you to directly cultivate and directly experience the Eight Extraordinary Channels. This book will begin to bridge the gap between the information in current texts on the Eight Extraordinary Channels, differing clinical applications from various traditions, and ancient insights of inner alchemy, personal development, and spiritual realization.

I hope you enjoy this book and find it beneficial in your cultivation and clinical practice.

Best wishes,
David Twicken
2012
Year of the Dragon

Qi Jing Ba Mai
Eight Extraordinary Channels

Qi

Qi can mean strange, wondrous, curious, extraordinary, or marvelous.

Jing

Jing can mean channel, vessel, meridian, and terrain. In this book, channels, vessels, and meridians are the same. These words are used interchangeably and refer to the pathways of the Eight Extraordinary Channels.

Ba

Ba is the number eight. There are eight channels/vessels. The number eight includes the eight directions, the source of all space and directions.

Mai

Mai can mean movement, animation, circulation, and pulsation in the channels.

THE CLASSICS AND THE EIGHT EXTRAORDINARY CHANNELS

There are many new archeological discoveries in China. As of now the oldest Chinese medical texts are from the Ma Wangdui tombs, which date to the Warring States period of the Zhou dynasty, 403–221 BC. The Han dynasty texts, *Su Wen* and *Ling Shu*, are considered the oldest Chinese medical texts that are part of the stream of knowledge commonly practiced today. The Eight Extraordinary Channels are not in the Ma Wangdui medical texts. They are presented in a scattered and brief way in the *Su Wen* and *Ling Shu*. Those two books are referred to as the *Nei Jing*. Six of the Eight Extraordinary Channels pathways are discussed in these early classics. The Yin Wei and Yang Wei have no pathway descriptions in the *Nei Jing*. The *Nei Jing* only states: "Yin Wei is where the Yin meets and the Yang Wei is where the Yang meets." *Su Wen* and *Ling Shu* have pathway descriptions for six of the Eight Extraordinary Channels. Yin Wei and Yang Wei channel pathways were not presented in those two books, but much later. There is only basic information for the other six channels in *Su Wen* and *Ling Shu*. Over time, more information has been added for all of the Eight Extraordinary Channels.

A later Han dynasty medical text is the *Nan Jing*. This text provides a little more detail and is more organized than the *Nei Jing*. The Wei channels' pathways and points are not described in the *Nan Jing*.

In the Jin dynasty, two major books were written. The first was the *Pulse Classic*. Wang Shu-he wrote it in 280 AD. This text includes pulses for the Eight Extraordinary Channels. The second book was the *Systematic Classic of Acupuncture and Moxibustion*. This book was written by Huang Fu Mi, and was completed in 282 AD. It is also called the *ABCs of Acupuncture*. The book is very interesting. It organizes the material of the *Su Wen*, *Ling Shu*, and other sources in a textbook format. The book has two sections that include the Eight Extraordinary Channels. Book II, Chapter 2, "The Eight Extraordinary Vessels," is similar to the *Su Wen* and *Ling Shu*. Book III contains the points on the primary channels, presented by regions of the body. The chapters describing the primary channel points indicate the Eight Extraordinary Channels points, including the Wei channels points. For the first time the Wei channels points are identified, but their pathways are not presented. This discrepancy is interesting. There is no original text from the Jin dynasty. The book was restored at a later time. This opens up the possibility that information was added to the text at a future time. The confluent (opening) points of the Eight Extraordinary Channels are not identified in this text.

In the Yuan dynasty a major change occurred regarding the knowledge and applications of the Eight Extraordinary Channels. Dou Hanqing wrote the *Guide of Acupuncture Canon* in 1196 AD. He presented the eight confluent points. These points are also called the master, opening and command points. Until this time they are not mentioned in any texts. He offers no theory as to why these points were selected.

The Ming dynasty was an important time for the development of the Eight Extraordinary Channels. In 1578, Li Shi-Zhen wrote the most detailed book on the Eight Extraordinary Channels: *Study of the Eight Extraordinary Vessels*. He is one of the most famous Chinese medical doctors and made significant contributions to pulse and herbal medicine. His *Ben Cao* ("original herbal book") is the standard material, and is still used as the basis of all that is written on herbs. Li Shi-Zhen adds points, functions, and applications to the Eight Extraordinary Channels. In his book the Yin and Yang Wei pathways are listed and are the foundation for what is used today. He includes herbs and pulses for the Eight Extraordinary Channels in his book.

In 1601, Xu Feng wrote the *Great Compendium of Acupuncture*, the *Zhen Jiu Da Quan*. This Ming dynasty text presents the common coupled pairings of the Eight Extraordinary Channels, and their confluent points. He systematically describes the Eight Extraordinary Channels. The text was one of the most comprehensive books at the time. It presents protocols for using the Eight Extraordinary Channels that are now considered classic methods. It was at this time that the Eight Extraordinary Channels and the confluent points became more commonly used in clinical practice. During this time a shift occurs in Chinese medical thinking. The *Nourish the Yin School* becomes popular at this time. It is one of the four great schools of Chinese medicine. This school explores how to influence Jing, and how influencing Jing can influence the constitution. This exploration leads to more insights into the Eight Extraordinary Channels and their influence on our life.

From a historical perspective, information about the Eight Extraordinary Channels has accumulated over a thousand years. This book includes aspects of these channels that are not part of most current school curricula, as well as a detailed presentation of the Eight Extraordinary Channels pathways based on modern insights. This book includes points on the pathways that are not formally listed in standard texts, but are on the internal pathways. They are an important part of the clinical applications. Included in the pathway section are descriptions from the *Pulse Classic*, which provides a flavor of the changes that have occurred since the Jin dynasty.

CHINESE DYNASTIES

Dynasty	Years
Pre-historic period	
Yangshao	5000 BC
Longshan	2500 BC
Xia	2100–1600 BC
Historic period	
Shang	1600–1045 BC
Zhou	1045–221 BC
Western Zhou	1045–771 BC
Eastern Zhou	770–256 BC
Spring and Autumn Period	722–481 BC
Warring States Period	403–221 BC
Qin	221–206 BC
Han	206 BC–AD 220
Western Han	206 BC–AD 24
Eastern Han	25 AD–AD 220
Three Kingdoms	220–280
Jin (Western and Eastern)	265–420
Southern and Northern	420–589
Sui	581–618
Tang	618–907
Five Dynasties and Ten Kingdoms	907–960
Song	960–1279
Liao	916–1125
Jin	1115–1234
Yuan	1271–1368
Ming	1368–1644
Qing (Manchu)	1644–1911
Republic of China	1912–1949
People's Republic of China	1949–present

INTRODUCTION

Chinese philosophy and medicine are based on systems of correspondences (resonances). During the Zhou dynasty, especially the Spring and Autumn and the Warring States periods, the foundation for this system of relationships developed. With contributions from Wang Wen and the *I Ching*, Lao Zi and the *Tao Te Ching*, Zou Yan and the natural school of Yin–Yang and Five Phases, and the internal alchemy tradition that included Wei Po Yang and the *Zhou I Can Tong Qi*, the ancient insight of perceiving the connections between humanity and nature was revealed. The theories and principles would be refined for centuries.

This book is guided by the insight of the early Chinese philosophical and medical practitioners: that humanity is inseparable from nature. This view requires a multi-dimensional view of life and Chinese medicine. The traditional qualities and functions of the Eight Extraordinary Channels are presented in this book, as well as their psycho-emotional and spiritual qualities. This additional information reflects an understanding of the "three treasures": Heaven, Humanity, and Earth (the physical, mental/emotional, and spiritual). Including these three aspects of life allows the practitioner to have a deeper understanding of the influences on a person's life. The three treasures is a system of correspondence. It is a model for understanding the multi-dimensional nature of life.

China is one of the world's oldest and most diverse cultures. Through the long history of China, three great traditions developed which had a profound influence on China. The traditions are Taoism, Confucianism, and Buddhism. These traditions contain guiding principles for how the Chinese express their understanding of life. Each of the three great traditions offers a unique insight into humanity and its relationship to nature. The unity of humanity and nature is a central theme among the traditions. The *Su Wen* and the *Ling Shu*, the early Han dynasty medical classics, contain not only medical insights but insights on lifestyle, and how to attune to the natural rhythms of nature. Attuning allows us to be in harmony with all of life. It allows for the awareness of the inseparable nature of Heaven, Humanity, and Earth. This awareness or consciousness is the common experience among all spiritual traditions, and is the most fundamental aspect of our life. The *Su Wen* and *Ling Shu* both present aspects of life that prevent us from realizing and living from our fundamental nature. From this perspective, these two classic Chinese texts are guides to self-realization. They provide a roadmap to adjust and attune to what has always existed, and is always with us: our Yuan Shen (original spirit).

The three treasures are an essential aspect of Chinese and Taoist spiritual and medical systems. Chinese spiritual and medical books offer a way to understand the three treasures. The understanding includes how life interactions and experiences create imbalances within the physical, emotional, and spiritual areas of our life. They also include guidance to find balance from life experiences. The *Ling Shu* can be translated as the spiritual compass. The text is also a compass to navigate through the Eight Extraordinary Channels. It can be used to understand how life experiences and interactions can create imbalances and illness. It is also a guide that creates an awareness of them. And it offers ways to understand, change, and transform them, and our life.

The Chinese view nature and life as a process that moves through cycles. Humanity is a microcosm of nature. We also move through cycles of transformation and change. The Eight Extraordinary Channels are presented from this viewpoint: as a mirror image of human development and human life cycles. The Eight Extraordinary Channels also have cycles of development. When we are stuck in a cycle or are resistant to change, the Eight Extraordinary Channels provide an opportunity to release and understand the stagnation or blockage. Understanding creates awareness, and a chance to take conscious action to change. Awareness allows the opportunity for the natural expression of our intrinsic, free-flowing nature. That single activity, becoming aware, is the most significant process for realization of our original nature (spirit). The great physician Li Shi-Zhen expressed that to really understand the Eight Extraordinary Channels, one needs to cultivate them with Nei Dan (inner meditation/ inner cultivation). In this text, a method for cultivating these channels is presented. I have practiced Nei Dan meditation for over 25 years. Through direct experience these channels come alive. They are no longer a theory, but living energy fields reflecting our lives.

PART I

THE EIGHT EXTRAORDINARY CHANNELS IN CLINICAL PRACTICE

Chapter 1

THE ACUPUNCTURE CHANNEL SYSTEM

The acupuncture channel system contains a sequence of levels that can be easily visualized from an anatomical layer perspective. Each layer or channel system corresponds to specific aspects of the body and their corresponding Chinese medical substances and related pathologies. The pathways of the channel system provide pointers to the "sequencing" of the channels. For example, *superficial* channel layers deal with the exterior and the pathology related to it, and the *deep* channels influence interior conditions and chronic constitutional conditions. The following shows the acupuncture layering system. Each layer will treat pathologies at its corresponding level more effectively than one channel system treating all layers.

Wei level—superficial

sinew channels

connecting (luo) channels

primary channels

divergent channels

Eight Extraordinary Channels

Yuan level—deep

The insight of the layering or sequencing of the channel system is clearly presented in the *Nei Jing*. The following *Nei Jing* references express this layering system. The Eight Extraordinary Channels are at the deep layers of the body.

"In general, when a pathogen invades the body, it first enters the skin level. If it lingers or is not expelled it will travel into the micro luo. If not expelled it travels to the regular luo channels, if not expelled it then moves to the main channels and then the internal organs."

"This is the progression of the pathogen from the skin level into the organs."

Nei Jing Su Wen, Chapter 63

"It is said the illness may be on the hair level, the skin level, the muscle level, the level of channels, tendon level, bone and marrow level. When treating the hair level do not damage the skin level. If the illness is at the skin level do not damage the muscle level, if the illness is at the muscle level needling too deeply will damage the channel level. In illness of the tendons needling too deeply will damage the bone level, in illness of the bones needling too deeply will damage the marrow."

Nei Jing Su Wen, Chapter 50

"When needling the bone level, take care not to needle the tendon level. When needling the tendon level do not injure the muscles. When needling the muscles, do not injure the channels and vessels. When needling the skin, do not injure the flesh or muscles."

Nei Jing Su Wen, Chapter 51

The Eight Extraordinary Channels are the domain of Jing and Yuan qi. These channels and substances influence and reflect the deepest aspects of our life, including our constitution and chronic patterns. This book presents how to use these channels to treat Jing and Yuan level conditions.

Chapter 2

THREE-LAYER THEORY

An important energetic model in Chinese philosophy and medicine is San Qing, which means "the three pure ones." From an energetic viewpoint, it reflects the interaction of three forces. From a macro viewpoint, it is a way to view universal interactions—for example, the interactions in the celestial realm. Tai Chi terminology and theory brings this macro theory to practical applications in medicine. The Tai Chi circle contains the Yang force (white color), the Yin force (black color), and the centerline or Yuan force (center curving line), and represents a three-force energy field. Heaven–Human–Earth and *shen*–qi–Jing are examples of this trinity model. In Chinese medicine, an important medical model of this theory is the three-layer theory. The three layers are Wei, Ying, and Yuan.

Superficial layer

Wei

Ying

Yuan

Deep layer

In the three-layer model, conditions can be viewed based on these layers or levels. When making a diagnosis, consider where the pathogen is located. From an Eight Extraordinary Channels viewpoint, pathogens and conditions at the Yuan level would be treated with these channels (see Tables 2.1 and 2.2). For example, a person who has chronic asthma would be diagnosed with Lung and Kidney qi deficiency. This is a chronic condition that is at the deep level, the Yuan level. This level corresponds to the Eight Extraordinary Channels, and source qi. The treatment therefore includes the Eight Extraordinary Channels

TABLE 2.1 THREE COMMON ENERGETIC LAYERS

Yang force	Heaven	Yu Ching	third ancestry	**Wei layer**	upper Dan Tian	*shen*	superficial
Yuan force	Human	Shan Ching	second ancestry	**Ying layer**	middle Dan Tian	qi	middle
Yin force	Earth	Tai Ching	first ancestry	**Yuan layer**	lower Dan Tian	Jing	deep

TABLE 2.2 THREE LAYERS AND THE
ACUPUNCTURE CHANNEL SYSTEM

Wei	sinews, luo and divergent channels
Ying	primary channels
Yuan	divergent and Eight Extraordinary Channels

Yuan Shen (original spirit)

Chinese culture contains a variety of spiritual traditions. Each tradition includes insights that are the basis of its teachings and practices. One insight is that each person has a Yuan Shen (original spirit). Part of this insight is that the creator and creation are one, undivided whole. By experiencing one's Yuan Shen, the unity of life is realized; the inseparable nature of life is realized; the clarity of one's true nature is realized. By directly experiencing one's Yuan Shen, it becomes clear what Yuan Shen is not. This insight is essential to self-realization, health, happiness, and transformation. Acupuncture can have a profound influence on releasing attachments and imprints that prevent an individual from realizing Yuan Shen. And it can guide one's focus or attention on self-realization.

A diamond in the rough

"A diamond in the rough" is an image that illustrates how the process of self-realization can occur. Each person has a diamond. The diamond is the Yuan Shen. The rough includes the stresses, conditioning, imprints, patterns, emotions, and unfavorable influences that exist in our life. We all have a diamond shining within, and we all have rough edges. The level and types of rough vary among people. Acupuncture can assist in releasing, clearing, and removing the rough. Acupuncture can clear away the rough, allowing insight and alignment with the diamond, which can be life changing. This insight can provide the inspiration and motivation to change a life, to live in a way that allows synchronization with *shen*, to be a living expression of *shen*. This is a way acupuncture can influence one's spirit. The knowledge of the channels, points, and energy centers allows the practitioner to develop customized treatments to treat the unique roughness of each person.

Chinese medicine includes a unique understanding of the psychological and spiritual aspects of a person's life. Chapter 5 of the *Su Wen*, "The Manifestation of Yin and Yang from the Macrocosm to the Microcosm," presents the five *shen*. These *shen* are a model for understanding patterns of disharmony. The five *shen* are the *shen*, *yi*, *po*, *zhi*, and *hun*, and they relate to the Heart, Spleen, Lungs, Kidneys, and Liver. *Shen* is Yang, and the five organs are Yin. The ancients viewed the Yin organs as housing the *shen*; Yang must have a Yin to contain it. The conditions of the *shen* can influence the Yin organs, and the conditions of the Yin organs can influence the *shen*. The *shen* relate to the five Yin organs and their correspondences.

Each *shen* has specific psychological qualities, and are used to match to their corresponding organ and channel. They provide a way to identify which organ and channel system is imbalanced and should be treated. Nei Dan and qi gong traditions offer many insights into the five *shen*.

Each of the five *shen* has unique corresponding emotions that reflect their condition. The following are key emotions (qualities) for each of the five *shen*:

- Hastiness, impatience, arrogance, cruelty, and hatred correspond to the Heart *shen*. Joy and love are the natural virtues.

- Worry, repetitive thinking, obsessive behavior, and jealousy correspond to the Spleen *yi*. Openness is the natural virtue.

- Sadness, depression, loneliness, isolation, and the inability to forgive correspond to the Lung *po*. Courage and righteousness are its natural virtue.

- Fear corresponds to the Kidney *zhi*, and gentleness is the natural virtue.

- Anger, irritability, and frustration correspond to the Liver *hun*, and kindness is the natural virtue.

When these emotions are imbalanced, match the emotion to the *shen* and organ, and treat their corresponding channels. In the model of the diamond in the rough, imbalances of these emotions are the rough. Acupuncture can assist in clearing the roughness, revealing the shining light of the diamond, the Yuan Shen. The Eight Extraordinary Channels provide a way to support the clearing of the roughness, releasing chronic and old patterns of roughness and redirecting a person to their diamond. Union with Yuan Shen can inspire, motivate, and provide the impetus for change and transformation.

Chapter 3

THE THREE ANCESTRIES

The Eight Extraordinary Channels can be viewed from a variety of perspectives. One view is cycles of life, an example of which is the cycles of seven and eight years presented in Chapter 1 of the *Su Wen*, "The Universal Truth." These cycles reflect changes that men and women move through during a lifetime. The cycles and transformations present with physical conditions, and also include emotional, psychological and spiritual changes. I refer to physical conditions as the first dimension, psycho-emotional conditions as the second dimension, and spiritual conditions as the third dimension. This book presents the three dimensions for applying the Eight Extraordinary Channels in clinical practice and Nei Dan.

The Chinese view change and process as an essential aspect of life. They perceive our life as containing three ancestries. Rooted in San Qing theory, the three ancestries is a way to view the Eight Extraordinary Channels from three major interactions or energetic formations. These channels unfold as our life unfolds, and this unfolding is seen in the three ancestries.

The first ancestry

The first ancestry is the Chong, Ren, and Du channels. This ancestry includes prenatal influences and early postnatal interactions. The first ancestry's energetics and imprints influence us throughout our lifetime. This is primarily the first cycle of our life. These cycles can be the seven- and eight-year cycles in Chapter 1 of the *Su Wen*, or the ten-year cycles in Chapter 54 of the *Ling Shu*, "The Allotted Year of a Man's Life."

The second ancestry

The second ancestry includes the Wei channels. It also includes our responses to life during cycles. The Wei channels allow us to understand our responses to life experiences as we move through cycles of time. They are a way to evaluate whether we are stuck in time. We can be stuck in past experiences or stresses with regard to the future. Wei channels can treat patterns set in the first ancestry, which can become patterns and imprints that are experienced during any time in a life. They can be life experiences or internal conflicts that create imbalances. The Wei channels are a way to access, influence, and treat patterns, imprints, and conditioning. Wei channels link to imbalances from Yin and Yang, form and action, and the past and future. The Wei channels can link to the first and third ancestries. They can release current intensities and assist the root of a condition.

The third ancestry

The third ancestry includes the Qiao and Dai channels. One function of the Qiao channels is as a reservoir, similar to luo channels. They contain or hold pathologies and can release them. To work on underlying patterns after a release, treat the Chong, Ren, and Du channels. Those channels influence the patterns and imprints that contain the root of the condition. When there is a crisis or an acute influence, with its root in a past experience, or thoughts or pressures of the future, consider the Qiao or Dai channels to release them. Between acute conditions, treat the first ancestry to address the root condition.

The Dai channel is the belt channel and it holds pathologies, including emotions. The Dai channel has the capacity to release pathogens and emotions we hold. Like undoing a belt and letting the abdomen out, the Dai channel allows things we hold to be let out. The Dai is a common channel to release the intensity of a condition and to prepare for working at a deeper level.

Unfolding of the three ancestries

Jing unfolds initially into the Chong, Ren, and Du channels. These channels are the predominant channels active during early human development.

Jing contains our genetic code, and initially unfolds into the Chong channel. From an acupuncture channel viewpoint, this is the origin of the channel system. The Chong channel is the most active channel *in utero*.

At birth the Ren channel is most active. The bonding process begins along the Ren channel when the mother/father/caretaker embraces the newborn. The baby connects first with their mother, belly to belly, mouth to mouth, eye to eye, mouth to nipple, Ren to Ren. This relationship has a profound influence on the child in all spheres of life: physical, emotional, and spiritual. The child falls in love with their caretaker. They fall in love with that person's emotional and energetic condition. They may seek that condition in their relationships in the future, whether it is favorable or unfavorable. Pathologies along the Ren can manifest later in life, depending on the bonding process. For example, if there was a lack of bonding, a person may seek that experience in future relationships. This type of bonding creates patterns that last until we consciously change them.

The Du channel becomes more active when a baby lifts its head and begins to explore its external environment. A lack of development of the Du channel may create someone who holds back, lacking the Yang motivation to look or move forward, and to interact with others. Too much stimulation of the Yang/Du channel can contribute to a person who must always be on the go, never stopping, full of Yang, and can't really slow down and enjoy just being in the moment. They view slowing down as a disturbing and unfavorable experience.

The Yang Wei and Yin Wei channels link different transitions or milestones in our life. People can invest their qi, blood, and essence (Jing) in reliving past moments or living a fantasy of the future. Being out of the present moment can be draining. The Wei channels can assist in releasing these attachments. These include how we respond to significant events and experiences during cycles of time.

The Yang and Yin Qiao channels relate to our stance in life. If a person is not clear about where they stand in life, which includes how they relate to the internal (self-esteem) or the external world (society), there can be imbalances that influence the Qiao channels. These are about the current moment. They offer the possibility of releasing or diminishing current intensities influencing our life.

The Dai channel is the belt channel and it is like a closet. It is where we store or stuff experiences that we cannot process or deal with in the current moment. If we do not deal with them in the future, the belt and closet fill up. If they are not resolved within a reasonable time, the body may not be able to hold them, and they can leak. Leakages can be body fluids, qi, blood, and Jing. The accumulations can be physical or emotional, visible or invisible. Treating the Dai channel opens the closet and cleans it out. The Dai channel is a means of releasing excesses and intensities, and is often used in initial treatments to release or let go. It provides a way to release the rough.

The three ancestries reveal how the Eight Extraordinary Channels function and interact. Figure 3.1 illustrates the unfolding of the Eight Extraordinary Channels.

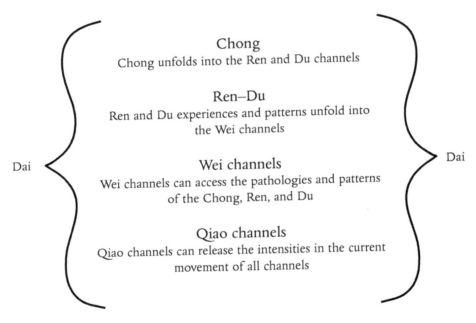

Dai

Chong
Chong unfolds into the Ren and Du channels

Ren–Du
Ren and Du experiences and patterns unfold into the Wei channels

Wei channels
Wei channels can access the pathologies and patterns of the Chong, Ren, and Du

Qiao channels
Qiao channels can release the intensities in the current movement of all channels

Dai

The Dai channel can release pathology in all channels

Figure 3.1 The unfolding of the Eight Extraordinary Channels

Unfolding of the Eight Extraordinary Channels

The Chong channel contains our prenatal, genetic, and ancestral influence. It is the life code that drives our development. It is the predominant channel functioning *in utero* and the first period of life. In postnatal life, experiences that are repetitive or intense can enter into the Yuan or Chong channel level. Postnatal influences and activities that are repeated can enter the Jing and become part of the constitution.

Source qi (Yuan qi) is Jing in qi form. Chong energetic properties are Jing in channel form. Jing is the root of Yin and Yang. Energetic properties of the Chong can unfold into the Yin and Yang channel system. Chong unfolds into the Ren channel. Yin pathology can unfold from the Ren to the Yin Wei and Yin Qiao. One image is to view them as interconnected: their influences can flow back and forth, and each channel can accesses and influence each other. This is prenatal influencing postnatal and postnatal influencing prenatal. This same dynamic functions for the Yang channels.

If there are Yin conditions, consider the Yin channel network to evaluate and treat. If there are Yang conditions, consider evaluating the Yang channel network. For example, if there is a Yin condition, a bonding or Yin deficiency, consider the Ren, Yin Wei, and Yin Qiao channels and evaluate them. Yin pathology can flow through the Yin channel network. The same applies to the Yang channel network. The pathology can move through its Yin or Yang network. This flow is a guide to using these channels as a diagnostic tool. It is a framework for asking questions related to each channel to make a clear diagnosis.

The Dai channel is the only horizontal channel, hence the "belt channel." It can be viewed as both Yin and Yang, and can influence all channels, especially excesses in all the channels. It connects left to right, and the lower to upper areas of the body.

Imbalances can transfer from the Yin to the Yang channel network, and the Yang to Yin channel network. A complete intake and diagnosis identifies the origin and branch of imbalances. Imbalances of Yin influence Yang and imbalances in Yang influence Yin. This relationship must be included in understanding the nature of a condition. It allows for understanding the root and branch of a condition.

Chapter 4

INTRODUCTION TO THE EIGHT EXTRAORDINARY CHANNELS

The Eight Extraordinary Channels encompass a wide range of qualities and functions. Traditional and non-traditional theories and functions are presented in this book, including theory, pathways, traditional functions, and psycho-emotional conditions.

The history of the Eight Extraordinary Channels is very interesting. In the *Su Wen* and *Ling Shu*, there are no pathway descriptions or points for the Wei channels. Their information was introduced at a later time. Most of the psycho-emotional, spiritual, and alchemical influences come from traditions not part of the common literature in the Chinese medical community.

It is believed that the Eight Extraordinary Channels confluent (opening) points were revealed by Dou Hanqing, in 1196 AD. He presented no theory to support their selection, and for this reason some practitioners do not use these points. They would always use the points on the Eight Extraordinary Channels pathways (trajectories), and might include the confluent points. Before Dou Hanqing the confluent points were not part of any known Chinese medical texts or traditions.

The legendary Xu Feng worked with the Eight Extraordinary Channels and made their applications popular in the Ming dynasty. Xu Feng did not always use the confluent points. He emphasized pathway points. Feng presented the common coupled pairs listed in Table 4.1, which have become the standard method of treatment. He did not always use those pairs. He used combinations that fit the diagnosis and treatment plan.

TABLE 4.1 XU FENG'S EIGHT EXTRAORDINARY CHANNEL PAIRS

Paired channels	Opening point	Regions affected when paired (traditional viewpoint)
Ren Yin Qiao	Lung 7 Kidney 6	Abdomen, chest, lungs, throat, face
Du Yang Qiao	Small Intestine 3 Bladder 62	Back of legs, back, spine, neck, head, eyes, brain
Chong Yin Wei	Spleen 4 Pericardium 6	Inner leg, abdomen, chest, heart, stomach
Dai Yang Wei	Gallbladder 41 San Jiao 5	Outer leg, sides of body, shoulders, sides of neck

Alternate names for confluent points are the command, opening, and master points.

- Four of the opening points are luo points: Lung 7, Spleen 4, Pericardium 6, and San Jiao 5.

- Two of the opening points are stream points: Small Intestine 3 and Gallbladder 41.

- Two of the opening points are at the beginning of their channel: Kidney 6 and Bladder 62.

- One pair is Tai Yang: Small Intestine 3 and Bladder 62.

- One pair is Shao Yang: Gallbladder 41 and San Jiao 5.

- One pair is Tai Yin: Lung 7 and Spleen 4.

- One pair can be considered Shao Yin: Kidney 6 and Pericardium 6.

Fundamental qualities of the Eight Extraordinary Channels

1. The Eight Extraordinary Channels regulate and influence cycles of seven and eight years from the *Su Wen*, or ten-year cycles from the *Ling Shu*, Chapter 54, "The Allotted Year of a Man's Life."

2. They store, distribute, and regulate vital substances (especially Jing and source qi) throughout the entire body.

3. They control the functions of the 12 primary channels.

4. They are closely related to the Kidneys, Gallbladder, and the Extraordinary Fu organs (Curious organs).

5. The Ren and Du channels have their own points. The other six channels borrow points from the 12 primary channels. The Kidneys and Gallbladder have the most Eight Extraordinary Channels points on their pathways.

6. The Eight Extraordinary Channels have no organs of their own. There is a strong link between the Curious organs and the Eight Extraordinary Channels. The Gallbladder is a link between the Curious organs, primary channels, and the Eight Extraordinary Channels.

7. Only the Ren and Du channels have connecting points.

8. Jiu Wei, Dove Tail, Ren 15, is the source point of the five Yin organs.

9. Each channel has a "confluent" point, which is also called the master, command, or opening point. They were revealed around 1196 AD, and popularized in the Ming dynasty. Classic acupuncture does not have these points.

10. Confluent points can be viewed as points that stimulate the Eight Extraordinary Channels pathways. Select points on the pathway to complete the stimulation of the channel. The pathway points send a clear message to the body that it is an Eight Extraordinary Channels treatment. Otherwise, how does the body know it is an Eight

Extraordinary Channels treatment, not a primary or a luo channel treatment (four confluent points are luo points)? Selecting points on the Eight Extraordinary Channels pathway directly probes and stimulates the channel's energetic properties. It is a key to an Eight Extraordinary Channels treatment.

11. Each channel has a common coupled paired channel, which is a creation in the Ming dynasty. Many practitioners combine paired points and channels based on diagnosis, not a fixed pairing. The channels can be paired in any way that fits the diagnosis.

12. The Wei and Qiao channels have cleft points. The Chong, Ren, Du, and Dai channels do not have cleft points. That implies that the Wei and Qiao channels are ways to clear stagnations or excesses. View these cleft points as ways to probe and stimulate flows throughout the channel. They are not just for pain. The Yang Wei has two cleft points: Bladder 63 is the Bladder cleft, and Gallbladder 35 is the cleft of the Yang Qiao.

13. The *Nei Jing* language primarily uses physical terminology when describing pathology. A unique insight of Chinese culture is that the body–emotions–spirit is an inseparable whole. It is for the practitioner to convert physical pathology and conditions to their corresponding emotional, psychological, and spiritual qualities. This book begins the process of revealing some of these relationships.

Chapter 5

THE CHONG CHANNEL

Common names

- Sea of Blood
- Yuan channel
- Thorough Way
- Penetrating channel
- Sea of the Twelve Regular Meridians
- Sea of Arteries and Veins

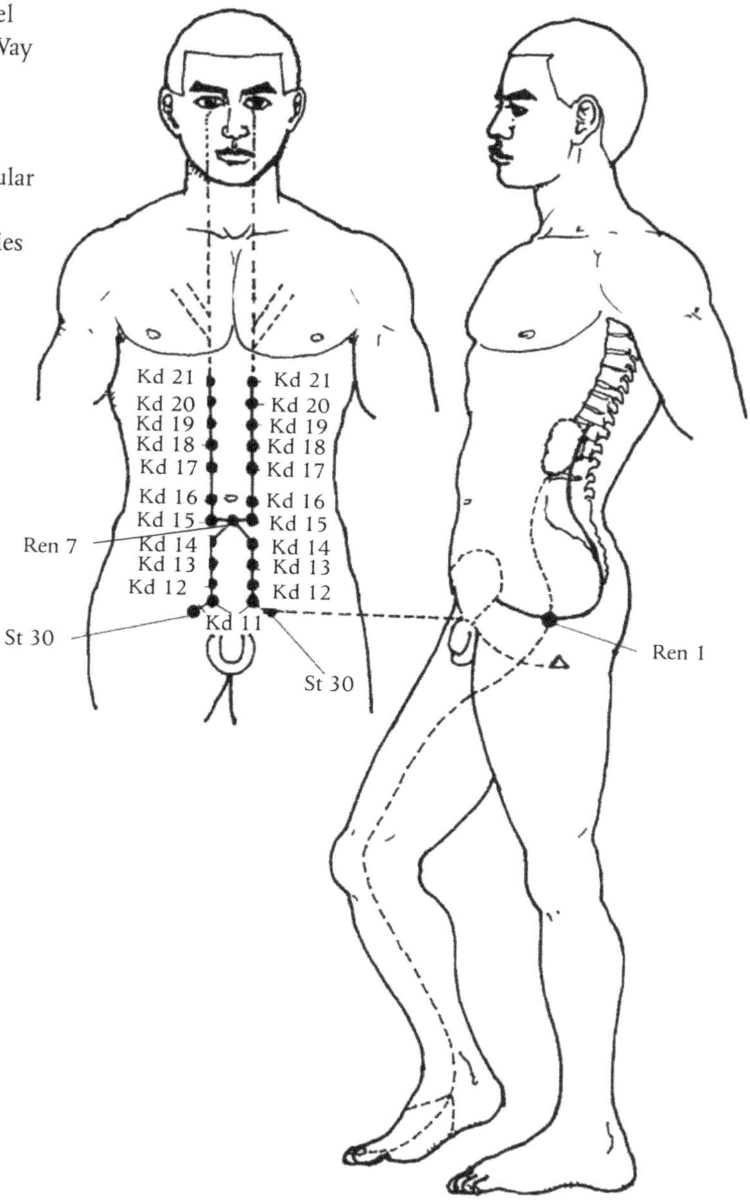

Figure 5.1 The Chong channel

The ancient Chinese accumulated knowledge by observing their external environment, the human body, and human behavior. This body of knowledge was applied to every area of life, including exercise, diet, astrology, feng shui, and the healing arts. The ancient Chinese perceived that life consisted of cycles, and that each cycle contained unique qualities and energetic properties. They were able to understand how the acupuncture channel system unfolded in cycles, and they understood that its unfolding was a mirror image of the unfolding of the universe.

In Chinese philosophy, the Tao is the origin of life. Tao is often called "the Way," the way of life. The Tao is the one all-pervading force. It is both the creator and creation. The Tao births Yin–Yang. Out of a single force, the Tao, a polarized force, is created. Yin–Yang is a polarized force that creates movement, interaction, and cycles. Yin–Yang differentiates. It contains a life code and force, to differentiate the body into organs, bones, muscles, glands, nerves, arteries, and veins. This unfolding of One/Tao, to the two/Yin–Yang, also occurs inside the human body. The Eight Extraordinary Channels illustrate this unfolding.

The Chong channel mirrors the energetic properties of the unfolding of the Tao. This single channel flows from the lower Dan Tian (behind and below the umbilicus) to Hui Yin, Ren 1, at the perineum, and flows up the front of the body, creating the Ren channel. It also flows from Hui Yin up the back of the body, to create the Du channel. This is the one creating the two. The Ren is the Sea of Yin, and the Du is the Sea of Yang.

The Tai Chi symbol reflects the first ancestry's unfolding. The curved line at the center is the Chong channel. It unfolds up the front of the body from the Yin position at the bottom. This is the Ren channel. It also flows from the Yin position up the back to create the Du channel. The Chong unfolds to create the Yin (Ren) and the Yang (Du) channels. The Chong will also unfold to create the Eight Extraordinary Channels. This unfolding is clearly presented in the pathway section that follows.

The value of knowing the unfolding of the Chong channel is that it creates all channels, and it can influence all of them. The Chong is both the origin and the branches of the Eight Extraordinary Channels. This is why needling any of the branches can influence the Chong channel's energetic properties. Combining channels and points in strategic combinations sends a clear message as to what channels and areas are targeted for treatment.

In Chinese medical theory, Jing or essence is the origin of the entire body. Jing is transformed into all substances and functioning. Jing transforms into the first energy in the body: source qi. It also transforms into the first channel: the Chong channel. From an energetic and channel perspective, the Chong channel is the unfolding of the genetic and destiny code contained in Jing.

Jing represents the self. The self is your core nature. This includes your genetics and ancestral lineage. If you do not like yourself, your ancestors or lineage, or desire to be someone else, you do not like your Jing or Yuan qi. This not liking creates a deep polarity and imbalance, which can manifest in all three dimensions (three treasures) in your life. Imbalances in the Chong channel can influence deep, core aspects of your life. Acceptance of self, ancestors, and genetics is the beginning of health and harmony. It dissolves a deep polarity. Acceptance does not mean following beliefs or behaviors that you disagree with; it means acknowledging realities of your life. Acknowledging can allow freeing up of unfavorable emotional attachments, and allow alternative ways of experiencing life free from the polarity. Experiencing life from a non-polarized and balanced state is living from present awareness, your natural condition—in other words, living from your spirit.

The Chong is very active in the first few years of life, during the first cycle of 7–8 years. It is most active *in utero*, and then the Ren becomes predominant until a child stands up and walks, when the Du channel becomes most active. The first few years of life are considered the most important in human development, which includes the influence of family and their culture and lifestyle. This influence includes the most influential imprints or conditioning on all channels and it has a profound effect on future behaviors and dynamics.

The Chong is responsible for moving or unfolding Jing. It unfolds Jing throughout the human body, which includes the channels, vital substances, organs, glands, bones, muscles, and tendons. The Chong moves Jing from prenatal to postnatal. The channel flows from the Kidneys to Qi Chong, Stomach 30. This is prenatal to postnatal, Kidneys to the Spleen, and Water to Earth.

The Chong channel connects Jing and *shen*, the Kidneys and the Heart. The channel begins in the lower Dan Tian, the Sea of Qi. The lower Dan Tian is where the Kidneys are located; there is a pathway that flows from there to the chest and the Heart. That connection reflects Jing seeking *shen*.

This channel or circuit is the built-in channel structure for each of us to seek and live from *shen* (spirit); this is our quest. The pathway also forms the front *shu* points. These points are Kidney 22–26, and relate to the five *shen*. This relationship shows we are built to seek, realize, and be an expression of our *shen*.

Chong energetic properties include the unfolding of Yin and Yang. Chong is the medium that allows us to connect and experience our prenatal nature, before the influences of people and society. The intensity of these influences and their capacity to take us away from our true nature can be viewed as influencing our spiritual condition. If the disconnect is too strong, we cannot live from this aspect of our spirit. An emotional condition can be viewed as floating in and out of a spirit connection. Floating out of it can be based on changing life situations. For example, meeting a person, or having to perform a certain role or task, can trigger an intense emotional response. When that person leaves, or the event is over, a more balanced condition occurs. The Chong channel offers a direct connection to our spiritual nature, our diamond, and offers the opportunity to become aware of it and to live from it.

In Chinese philosophy, the Tao births Wu Ji. In birthing Wu Ji, the process of creation is set in motion. The code of creation exists inside Wu Ji. The code includes the potentiality to become anything. Wu Ji is before Yin–Yang. Wu Ji is not shaped. Chong energetic properties can access our primordial nature, the capacity to become anything, to take any shape or form. This includes having an open and free mind. Culture or society can place limitations on us and try to shape us. They can try to limit how we view life, how we think and behave. A goal of personal development is to cultivate Jing and the Chong channel, allowing the unity of our body, mind and spirit, or our *shen*, qi, and Jing. This unity enables our daily life to become a natural expression of our true nature. This is a quest. This quest is the same for all people. The road and specific areas to cultivate vary depending on ancestral, genetic, cultural, family, and other postnatal influences.

In Chinese spiritual traditions, humanity is inseparable from nature. Their cultivation practices lead to this realization. When we realize we are part of nature, we see no difference between our self and nature. For example, when perceiving the sun, we *are* the sun, when perceiving the moon and the stars, we *are* the moon and the stars. This awareness is the ability to be all things. This is living from our Wu Ji nature.

The acupuncture point Gong Sun, Spleen 4, is on an Earth channel and is a luo point (blood point). Gong Sun is the opening point of the Chong channel. This is how Earth, or postnatal qi and blood, influences and shapes us. It is Earth shaping Water. It is the Spleen shaping the Jing of the Kidneys, by way of the Chong channel. Spleen 4 and the Earth channel influence our prenatal nature. The Spleen and Earth represent postnatal life and its influences. By cultivating our postnatal influences (our lifestyle), we influence the prenatal by adjusting the way postnatal influences prenatal. When we can allow the natural expression of our prenatal energetic properties in postnatal life, we are living our quest. This process is a type of alchemy. This cultivation influences the way we can change and transform. The Chong channel offers the capacity to reconnect and re-align to our Yuan Shen, our original spirit.

Significant pathway qualities of the Chong channel

The Chong channel has mostly Kidney points. There is a strong pathway connection between the Chong, the Kidneys and the Heart. These relationships show how the Chong channel influences the relationship of the Kidneys and Heart (Shao Yin), and Jing and *shen*.

The Chong supports the prenatal and postnatal. It supports the Stomach/Spleen and the Kidneys. The Chong internal pathway flows from the lower Dan Tian and moves to Qi Chong, Stomach 30, which is one of the Sea of Grain points. This pathway shows the strong connection between the Kidneys and Spleen, prenatal and postnatal. The Chong supports Earth and Earth shapes the prenatal. Treating Qi Chong can influence the Kidneys and the Stomach and Spleen. Because the Chong channel is the origin of all channels, it can support all organs. The other channels and points in the treatment determine which organs are being treated.

The Chong pathway is located in the area of Jing, the lower abdomen, and moves to the location of postnatal qi, the abdomen. This pathway is part of the first trajectory. The second pathway flows to the Heart and chest. These two trajectories show how Jing seeks *shen*.

- *The Chong channel births Yin (Sea of Yin) and Yang (Sea of Yang)*:

    ◦ Birthing Yin, the pathway forms the Sea of Yin, the Ren channel.

- ○ Birthing Yang, the pathway forms the Sea of Yang, the Du channel.

- *The Chong channel births the Dai channel.* The Chong channel begins in the lower abdomen and wraps around the back to the spine. This wrapping creates the Dai channel, the belt channel.

- *The Chong channel births the leg channels,* the Qiao and Wei channels. The pathway moves to the heels, including both the medial and the lateral malleolus. This pathway includes the Yin and Yang Qiao, and eventually the Wei channels.

- *The Chong channel is the Sea of Blood.* The Chong channel nourishes blood. Its pathway supports the Spleen, and creates the pathway and energy network that allows communication between the Kidneys, essence, blood, the Pericardium, and the Heart. This is a reason for the coupled pairing of Gong Sun, Spleen 4 and Nei Gong, Pericardium 6.

Internal pathway

The Chong channel's internal pathway consists of five branches.

First branch

The pathway begins in the lower abdomen, in the uterus for women, and emerges at the perineum, Hui Yin, Ren 1. The pathway:

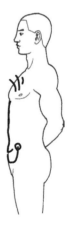

- influences the lower Dan Tian, source qi, Jing, and prenatal energetic properties

- influences the genitals and fertility

- is the origin of Chong, Ren, Du, and Dai channels.

Ascending, it runs inside of the spinal column. This is the creation of the Du channel.

The channel goes from the center, in the lower Dan Tian, to the back. This pathway implies the creation of the Dai channel.

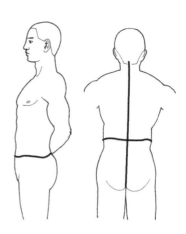

Second branch

The second branch flows from Hui Yin, Ren 1, passes through the region of Stomach 30, Qi Chong, and communicates with the Kidney channel at Kidney 11, Heng Gu. It then ascends throughout the Kidney channel to You Men, Kidney 21. The pathway then disperses in the chest. This pathway:

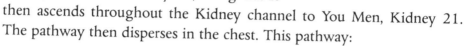

- influences the Stomach and Earth

- includes the lower, middle, and upper abdomen; including the chest, Lungs, and Heart

- supports postnatal qi: the Spleen, Stomach, and Lungs

- connects the Kidneys and Heart and Jing and *shen*

- influences the pubic bone; Jing is closely related to bone

- forms the front *shu* points: Kidney 22–26.

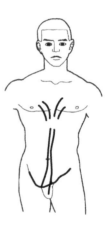

Third branch

From the chest, the third branch ascends alongside the throat, curves around the lips, and terminates below the eye. This is the end of the Ren channel.

This branch influences the throat, face, mouth, and eyes.

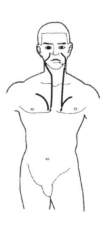

Fourth branch

The fourth branch emerges at Qi Chong, Stomach 30, and descends the medial areas of the legs to the popliteal fossa. It then descends the medial aspects of the lower legs and runs posterior to the medial malleolus, terminating on the sole (heel) of the foot.

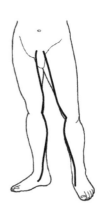

A branch descends obliquely to the malleolus towards the Stomach channel and enters the heel, and then crosses the tarsal of the foot. This pathway creates the Yin Qiao and Yin Wei channels, and:

- influences the Kidneys, Bladder, and Stomach channels

- treats cold in the lower limbs

- implies that the channel flows through Xue Hai, Spleen 10, Yin Gu, Kidney 10, and Wei Zhong, Bladder 40.

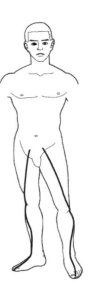

Fifth branch

From Qi Chong, Stomach 30, the pathway flows down to Chong Yang, Stomach 42, to the big toe. This pathway creates the Yang Qiao and Yang Wei channels.

This internal pathway flows past Chong Yang, Stomach 42, Tai Chong, Liver 3, Da Dun, Liver 1 and Yin Bai, Spleen 1. Note that the last three points are major blood points.

Anatomical areas of influence

Big toe, feet, legs, uterus, lumbar region, abdomen, chest, Heart, breasts, throat, face, head, Kidneys, and the genitals. Jing, Blood, and Yuan qi.

Common conditions the Chong channel treats

Regulates blood, infertility for males and females, impotence, gynecological conditions, irregular menses, blood-related conditions, colic, spasms, and pain in the abdomen, rebellious qi in the chest and abdomen, asthmatic breathing, rebellious Lung qi, dyspnea, counter-flow qi, running piglet, and atrophy disorders of the leg.

Chong channel points and functions

Ren 1   Hui Yin   Meeting of Yin

Meeting of the Chong and Du channels. Ghost point. Luo point.

DESCRIPTION

Hui Yin is the meeting of Yin, and it has a profound influence on Yin in the body. It is located in the lowest area of the lower Dan Tian and it influences this Dan Tian. In qi gong, this area is squeezed to stimulate and strengthen the local muscles and the energetic properties of the entire lower Dan Tian. Squeezing this area also influences the Du channel and the top of the head. It can stimulate the flow of qi up the Du channel and the Microcosmic Orbit, the circuit created by the Du and Ren channels. This gentle squeezing is the Deer Exercise, a type of qi gong practice. Ren 1 is used in Yin–Yang treatments. Bai Hui, Du 20 is at the vertex. Both points have Hui in their name and stimulating one of them stimulates the other point. Du 20 is often used to treat hemorrhoids. This area is connected to the Kidneys and influences Jing. The Chong, Ren, and Du channels meet at this point.

TREATMENT

Nourishes Yin, calms *shen*, clears damp heat in the lower Jiao, clears blockages in the lower Jiao, and regulates the genitals, anus, and sexuality. It can release chronic pathogens and trauma related to early life.

Ren 7   Yin Jiao   Yin Junction

Lower Dan Tian point.

DESCRIPTION

Yin Junction is a place where Yin can be gathered and influenced. It can influence Yin substances, channels, and conditions. Yin also refers to bonding. This point can assist a person in understanding bonding in their life. It can gather Yin substances in the body. It is a superb point to mobilize Yin and direct it to channels, organs, or areas of the body. Yin Junction is a powerful point to ground or root a person. Ren 7 is a major point for stimulating the lower Dan Tian. It is the lower Dan Tian point of the three Dan Tian points: Ren 17 for the upper Dan Tian; Ren 12 for the middle Dan Tian; and Ren 7 for the lower Dan Tian. It can influence the Kidneys and Jing.

TREATMENT

Influences all Yin: Yin, blood, fluids, phlegm, nodules, and fibroids. Regulates the uterus, moves damp, and regulates the lower Dan Tian.

Stomach 30   Qi Chong   Penetrating Qi

Sea of Grain point. Meeting of the Du and Ren channels.

DESCRIPTION

Qi Chong has a powerful relationship with the Kidneys, Jing, and source qi. It connects directly to prenatal energetic properties and our Yuan Shen. This point treats Yuan level conditions and has a powerful influence on moving one past stagnant conditions, which can be physical or psycho-emotional. Qi Chong is one of the most powerful points to reinforce prenatal and postnatal substances. It is a potent point to move blood, especially related to the menstrual cycle.

TREATMENT

Moves qi and blood in the Chong channel. Regulates the Chong channel. Promotes essence and treats infertility. Tonifies the Spleen and Stomach. Moves damp. Invigorates blood in the uterus. Subdues rebellious qi in the lower Dan Tian. This is one of the best points to tonify post- and prenatal substances.

Kidney 11   Heng Gu   Pubic Bone

Heng Gu is right off the pubic bone.

DESCRIPTION

Jing has a close relationship with bone and the marrow matrix: Jing, marrow, bone, spine, brain, and blood. Bone is part of the Kidney correspondences and this point treats the Kidneys, bone, and marrow issues.

TREATMENT

Urogenital and gynecological conditions. Influences the Kidneys, Jing, and bone.

Kidney 12   Da He   Great Manifestation

Da He is one cun above the pubic bone. It is where the Chong channel qi comes out from deep inside the body, the Yuan level. It is where the Chong's life code is unfolding in the postnatal area of the body.

DESCRIPTION

Great Manifestation can mean this point's ability to influence fertility, to create life, to give birth. This area is four cun below Shen Que, Ren 8, and is level with Ren 3, Zhong Ji, Central Pole. From a Taoist perspective, the Central Pole is the center of the body. It is the cosmic correspondence to the North Star, the Taoist center of the universe. Central pole can be used to ground and root a person in their center, Yuan, or original nature. Taoist traditions are center-based. Out of the center, life originates. By stimulating the center, life is birthed. In dimension one (the physical), Da He can be used along with other channels and points to manifest a new life. In dimension two (psycho-emotional), it can help attune a person to a new awareness and expression of their life. In dimension three (spiritual), it can realign a person to their *shen* and cosmic unity.

TREATMENT

Treats urogenital and gynecological conditions. Harmonizes the Heart–Kidney relationship. Panic attacks. Yin deficiency. A major fertility and conception point. Regulates the uterus and menses. Tonifies the Kidneys and essence.

Kidney 13   Qi Xue   Qi Hole   Uterine Gate

DESCRIPTION

Qi Hole is an area where the qi of the Kidneys can be guided out to support the Spleen, the postnatal. This point is level with Guan Yuan, Ren 4, which is a major reinforcing point. It also has a strong influence on the uterus. Use this point when using the Chong channel to support the Spleen. It also influences fertility.

TREATMENT

Treats urogenital, gynecological, and blood conditions. Supports the Spleen. Dawn conditions: cock's crow diarrhea, discharge, and turbid urine. Infertility. Consolidates the Ren and Chong. Running piglet.

Kidney 14   Si Man   Fourfold Fullness

DESCRIPTION

Fourfold Fullness can treat the four limbs. When there is fullness or damp in the four limbs, this point can help resolve damp. Si Man is most effective when the Kidneys are involved in the condition. Shi Man, Stone Gate, Ren 5 is the front *mu* of the San Jiao and a major moving and reinforcing point. Si Man is level with Shi Man and influences San Jiao energetics.

TREATMENT

Treats urogenital, gynecological, and blood conditions. Edema of the four limbs. Fluid accumulation in lower Jiao. Treats the Spleen. Nourishes essence and marrow.

Kidney 15   Zhong Zhu   Central Flow

Central Flow is level with Yin Junction, Ren 7.

DESCRIPTION

If one is not in a healthy flow in life, this point can help readjust and realign to a healthy flow, especially when the *zhi* and willpower is part of the condition. Taoist theory is center-based. By going to the center of our body or life, we can obtain balance and re-establish the natural flow in life.

TREATMENT

A major urination point. Urogenital, gynecological, and blood conditions. Constipation due to deficiency. Nourishes Kidney Yin.

Kidney 16   Huang Shu   Vital Membranes

Huang Shu is level with Shen Que, Ren 8 and the umbilicus.

DESCRIPTION

This is the upper end of the lower Dan Tian and directly affects Jing, the Gate of Vitality, and source qi. The Chong and Kidney channels have pathways that flow to the Heart. Huang Shu can treat Shao Yin or Kidney and Heart conditions. It can nourish the Heart with Yin, essence, and qi. Huang Shu influences the relationship of this area to the *shen*. It also influences the vital regions of the lower Dan Tian: Ming Men Fire, Gate of Vitality, Jing, Kidneys, and the Chong channel.

TREATMENT

Treats urogenital and gynecological conditions. Tonifies the Kidneys. Benefits Shao Yin and blood. Descends Lung qi to the Kidneys. Helps the Kidneys grasp Lung qi. Benefits the membranes surrounding organs. Regulates the intestines.

Kidney 17   Shang Qu   Shang Bend   Bent Metal

Shang Qu is just above Water Separation, Ren 9.

DESCRIPTION

When Water is ample, our body and life is fluid and we can adjust or bend to deal with life. This point can assist in becoming more flexible and able to adapt to conditions and interactions in life. Water Separation is about the Small Intestine's ability to separate the pure from the impure in our assessments, judgments, and decisions. Shang Qu can assist in being flexible in those actions, not rigid, stiff, and inflexible. Water's nature is to be fluid. It can adjust and adapt to any size or form. When Water is frozen its intrinsic nature is dissolved. Shang Qu assists in restoring the intrinsic nature of Water and our self.

TREATMENT

Strengthens the Kidneys and Spleen qi. Grasps Lung qi. Clears accumulations in the lower Jiao. Regulates the intestines.

Kidney 18   Shi Guan   Stone Pass

DESCRIPTION

Stone Pass contains an aspect of the Chong channel's surging function. This point is between the lower and middle Dan Tian. It can influence the Chong's ability to move and surge its energy and influence into the middle Dan Tian. This point can assist in breaking through stones, which can mean phlegm, damp, accumulations, and emotional blockages. It also assists in passing through blockages of ancestral influences of the Kidneys and the *zhi*, and the postnatal influences of the Spleen, Stomach, and *yi*. Zhong Wan, Ren 12, is the front *mu* of the Stomach. Stone Pass can assist in helping one pass from ancestral to postnatal influences. This is Jing and qi influences in the *shen*–qi–Jing transformation process. This passing is necessary to make a clear connection to the *shen* center at Tan Zhong, Ren 17.

TREATMENT

Resolves phlegm, moves blood, treats constipation, supports Kidney qi to ascend.

Kidney 19   Yin Du   Yin Metropolis

DESCRIPTION

A metropolis is a meeting place. Here, it is a meeting of Yin qualities. It is Yin in the Yang. The Yang is the upper portion of the body. Ren 1 to Ren 7 are Yin within Yin. Yin includes grounding, rooting, nourishing, supporting, loving, and bonding. Level with Zhong Wan, Ren 12, the front *mu* of the Spleen, the Earth element contains the Yin qualities of grounding, rooting, centering, calming, and nourishing. Yin Du can influence Spleen and *yi* conditions. If the *yi* is imbalanced and there is worry, too much thinking, especially repetitive thinking, this point can assist in focusing the *yi* into the center. It can assist in applying one's will to move to the center. The center dissolves an imbalanced *yi*. And it opens one to the spontaneity of life, not fixed, rigid patterns of the past. To be in the center is to be in the present moment. The present moment is an awareness of the Earth element's energetics. Yin Du especially treats *yi* imbalances due to Kidney, willpower, and *zhi* imbalances. Yin Du can gather, collect, and guide Yin. It has functions similar to Yin Jiao, Ren 7.

TREAMENT

Clears mucus. Nourishes blood. Treats infertility due to blood stagnation. Yin Du can be used for disharmony of Shao Yin, the Heart, and the Kidneys.

Kidney 20   Fotong Gu   Abdomen Connecting Valley Open Valley

DESCRIPTION

An open valley allows a free flow. This point assists in allowing the flow of the Chong channel from the middle Dan Tian, the Spleen/Stomach and *yi*, to the Heart *shen*. If ancestral and postnatal influences from our actions in life have diminished our faith in life, this point can help develop our faith to achieve our inner purpose. Fotong Gu stimulates the Chong channel's moving function, creating a smooth flow like Water flowing in a river. It assists in the Chong's quest for self-realization.

TREATMENT

This point supports the Spleen's ability to ascend its qi to the Lungs. It influences Gu qi and blood.

Kidney 21   You Men   Dark Gate

DESCRIPTION

The Chong channel begins in the most Yin part of the body, the lower Dan Tian, the Kidneys, and the uterus. In this darkness or Yin, light and life is created. You Men is level with Great Tower, Ren 14, the front *mu* point of the Heart. You Men is a gate to the Heart. The Chong pathway flows to You Men, and then disperses into the chest and to the front *shu* points. When there are issues that prevent one from connecting to their Heart *shen*, or one is unable to live from their Heart, this point can assist in clearing these blockages. When fear or phobias prevent growth and transformation, consider You Men. Alchemy is transforming darkness to light, dense to subtle, and Jing to *shen*. You Men assists in this process.

TREATMENT

Harmonizes the Stomach. Descends Stomach turbidity. Opens the Kidneys and the *zhi* to allow the Heart to descend and communicate. Clears Heart heat. Moves qi and blood. Moves qi in the chest.

Front *shu* points

The Chong pathway spreads around the chest. The pathway ranges from Kidney 22–27, and includes the front's five *shu* points: Kidney 22–26. The five front *shu* points correspond to the five Yin organs and the five *shen*. They can be used to treat the organs, as well as their psycho-emotional qualities.

Kidney 22   Bu Lang   Corridor Walk   Step Gallery

- Corresponds to Kidney *shu*, *zhi*, Water, Kidneys.
- This is the front *shu* of the Kidneys and treats the *zhi*.
- Fifth intercostal space.

Kidney 23   Shen Feng   Spirit Seal

- Corresponds to Spleen *shu*, *yi*, Earth, Spleen.
- This is the front *shu* of the Spleen and treats the *yi*.
- Fourth intercostal space.

Kidney 24   Ling Xu   Spirit Ruins

- Corresponds to Liver *shu*, *hun*, Wood, Liver.
- This is the front *shu* of the Liver and treats the *hun*.
- Third intercostal space.

Kidney 25   Shen Cang   Spirit Storehouse

- Corresponds to Heart *shu*, *shen*, Fire, Heart.
- This is the front *shu* of the Heart and treats the *shen*.
- Second intercostal space.

Kidney 26   Yu Zhong   Lively Center

- Corresponds to Lung *shu*, *po*, Metal, Lungs.

- This is the front *shu* of the Lungs and treats the *po*.

- First intercostal space.

Confluent point (command, opening, master point)

- Gong Sun, Yellow Emperor, Spleen 4.

- Luo point of the Spleen.

Coupled point

- Nei Gong, Inner Gate, Pericardium 6.

- Luo point of the Pericardium.

Chapter 6

THE REN CHANNEL

Common names

- Conception channel
- Controlling channel
- Directing channel
- Sea of Yin
- Sea of Bonding
- Sea of Relationships
- Responsibility channel
- Channel of Synchronicity

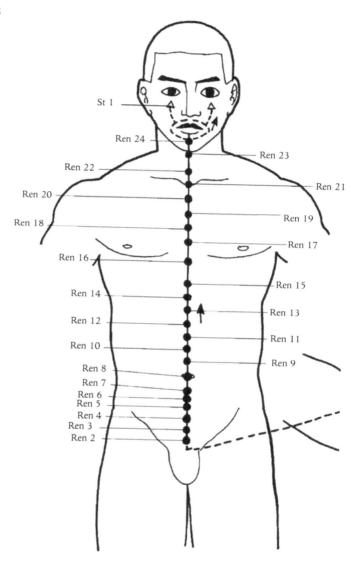

St 1

Ren 24

Ren 22

Ren 20

Ren 18

Ren 16

Ren 14

Ren 12

Ren 10

Ren 8

Ren 7

Ren 6

Ren 5

Ren 4

Ren 3

Ren 2

Ren 23

Ren 21

Ren 19

Ren 17

Ren 15

Ren 13

Ren 11

Ren 9

Figure 6.1 The Ren channel

The Ren channel comprises and influences the Yin of the body. The Yin of the body includes the bones, muscles, tendons, organs, blood, fluids, and Jing. The Ren channel includes the nature or condition of these Yin substances. The Ren is Yin, which corresponds to bonding, especially how we bond to our parents and family.

The Chong births Ren. *In utero* we are undifferentiated from our mother and we are influenced by her condition. This includes her physical, emotional, and spiritual condition. After birth we bond with our caretakers. I will refer to this person as "mom" for convenience; it can be dad or a caretaker. We are influenced by all of them, especially when we are held. We bond belly–belly, mouth–mouth, eye–eye and mouth–nipple. The newborn is sensing, feeling, touching, and listening to mom, similarly to *in utero*. Bonding includes all aspects of smelling, feeling, and touching. Mom's condition transfers to the newborn.

The child physically bonds to the front of their mom's body. It is caressed and cradled from the front, which is Yin. This bonding area of the body is the Ren channel pathway. The child seeks nourishment from food, as well as the energy of, and connection to, the people in the child's life. The baby receives imprints of types of bonding that include mom's physical, emotional, and spiritual condition. There is a transfer from the caretaker to the child. The bonding received can be an excess or deficiency. The nature of the bonding contributes to imprints or images that influence a person throughout a lifetime. These imprints can influence our emotions and behavior patterns in our relationships in the future.

The early imprints can be what we seek later in life when we desire nourishment or nurturing. We seek to connect with others who have those early imprints. As we look at our relationships and the way we bond with our partners, friends, and family, consider Ren channel treatments for imbalances in those areas of life.

Bonding includes the mouth, because it is on the Ren channel. Di Cang, Stomach 4, is located at the corner of the mouth and can be influenced by the bonding process. The process can influence our relationship to food. To what degree is our eating behavior driven by emotions or psychological influences? Understanding the bonding process can help understand and change some eating habits.

Bonding includes a feeling of being united with others. It includes the feeling of belonging and being accepted by others. The type of bonding that occurs early in life can be the cause of behaviors later in life. Included in the bonding process is the desire for wholeness, to be united, to be complete. We seek bonding based on our experiences in life. If our relationships do not bring the nurturing and nourishment desired, consider the bonding process presented to understand their origin. This knowledge can be a guide to understanding choices in relationships, and the basis for changing the patterns.

Consciousness of the bonding process and identifying patterns related to it brings the opportunity to take actions that can lead to change. Using our willpower, or *zhi*, to synch or bond with different aspects of life, holds the seeds for transformation. Qi gong and meditation allow for bonding to different aspects of life, different rhythms, and different vibrations. We can cultivate ourselves to bond or synch to our Yuan Shen, our original nature, and with the Tao.

There can be a Ren excess condition. Ren excess can be a condition of overly bonding. Maybe the child was smothered, controlled, and prevented from interacting with other people. If this occurs a child can become overly dependent and do things to further the dependency. This pattern can lead to dependency and actions to maintain the dependency. If this condition exists, consider evaluating Ren energetic properties and doing Ren treatments.

Too much bonding can mean too much Yin. The Yin is in excess, which is an accumulation. The accumulation can allow one to feel fulfilled, but the accumulation is stagnation. It is the body trying to hang on to something, to maintain something. Stagnations can include damp, phlegm, fibroids, masses, or tumors. The desire to resolve this stagnation, to let go of what one is trying to maintain, is necessary to allow space for change. Acupuncture will not transform it alone. Qi gong, herbs, guidance, etc., may be needed to assist in this change.

Lack of bonding is a Yin deficiency. One may not feel content or complete, or may be unable to feel happy or satisfied in daily life. This Yin deficiency can cause dryness, emptiness, and empty heat. Ren treatments may assist in enabling one to feel happy, content, and nourished. Placing a needle in a body is felt as receiving, connecting, and bonding. Some patients request or demand more needles in a treatment; this can indicate their desire to feel nourished.

Ren energetic properties include identifying with the early influences in our life. The influences include family, friends, culture, and society. Family and their religious, political, and life viewpoints are the first things introduced in a child's life; they contribute to the conditioning that occurs. These influences can create imprints that exist for a lifetime. Understanding the root of the condition allows for a clear treatment plan, including which Eight Extraordinary Channels to select. A model for evaluating where these influences manifest is the three Dan Tian.

The three Dan Tian

Dan Tian means "energy field." There are three Dan Tian. They include the lower, middle, and upper areas of the body.

The *lower* Dan Tian includes the area from Hui Yin, Ren 1, up to around Shen Que, Ren 8. This Dan Tian includes the area where human life is created: the uterus. It also includes the first Dan Tian, the first acupuncture channel: the Chong channel, and the first points in the body. This center includes the Kidneys, Jing, genitals, and fertility. The lower center includes prenatal and ancestral influences. This area and its points correspond with the first influences in our life. When there are conditions related to these areas of life, consider the lower Dan Tian for treatment.

The *middle* Dan Tian relates to transformation. The middle Dan Tian ranges from about Shen Que, Ren 8, to Jiu Wei, Ren 15. This Dan Tian corresponds to transforming, controlling, and shaping. The need to be in control is related to the Spleen/Stomach and *yi*. The energetic properties of this Dan Tian include the consequences of our actions—the karma we have created. When there are conditions related to our choices and actions in life, consider the middle Dan Tian for treatment.

The *upper* Dan Tian ranges from around Jiu Wei, Ren 15, to Bai Hui, Du 20. This Dan Tian corresponds to the Heart center. This center relates to love, spiritual clarity, and realization. A hug is a connection to this center. A hug is an expression of love, which is within every person. If someone has lost the ability or desire to love, consider the upper Dan Tian in a treatment strategy.

Each of the three centers/the three Dan Tian relates to areas and influences in our life. The lower Dan Tian relates to ancestral influences, the middle Dan Tian relates to our own actions and their conditions, and the upper Dan Tian relates to love, spiritual clarity, and realization. Imbalances in one Dan Tian can influence the others. For example, prenatal and early life influences can influence how we interact in postnatal life.

Breakthrough in one Dan Tian can assist in transforming imbalances in the other Dan Tian. Identifying where a person may be stuck or having challenges provides the clinician with a model to assist in bringing awareness of the condition and the opportunity for change.

Internal pathway

The Ren channel's internal pathway consists of four branches.

First branch

The Ren channel begins below Zhong Ji, Central Pole, Ren 3, or in the uterus for females and in the lower abdomen for males. The pathway emerges at the perineum, Hui Yin, Ren 1. This branch influences the lower Dan Tian, genitals, fertility, gynecology, Jing, and the Kidneys.

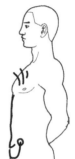

Second branch

The branch ascends along the midline of the abdomen, chest, throat, and jaw. It terminates at Cheng Jiang, Ren 24. It influences the organs in the local area and six front *mu* points on the Ren channel.

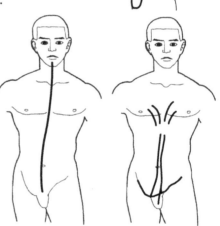

Third branch

The interior portion of the channel winds around the mouth and then connects with the Du channel at Yin Jiao, Gum Intersection, Du 28. It curves around the lips and terminates below the eye at Cheng Qi, Stomach 1. It influences the throat, face, and eyes.

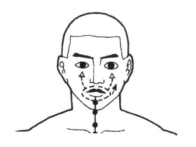

Fourth branch

This branch arises in the pelvic cavity, enters the spine and ascends along the back. This pathway is the Du channel.

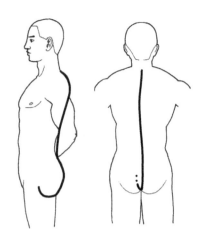

The Ren pathway according to the Pulse Classic

Originates from the Bao Men, Uterine Gate, and travels upward to the umbilicus and reaches the chest. It is said in another version that the conception originates from Zhong Ji, Central Pole, Ren 3, rises to the pubic hair region, proceeds inside the abdomen up through the Guan Yuan, Origin Pass, Ren 4, and ends in the throat.

Anatomical areas of influence

The Ren channel influences the genitals, uterus, abdomen, lower Jiao, thorax, Heart, Lungs, throat, face, and eyes. It influences the reproductive system, menstruation, fertility, pregnancy, and menopause. It controls all Yin: Jing, blood, fluids, damp, and phlegm.

Common conditions the Ren channel treats

Stagnations in the lower Jiao, especially genital and urinary conditions. Nourishes Yin and essence. Calms *shen*. Treats vaginitis, enuresis, nocturnal emission.

Ren channel points and functions

Ren 1   Hui Yin   Meeting of Yin

Ghost point. The meeting of the Chong and Du channels.

DESCRIPTION

Hui Yin is the meeting of Yin and has a profound influence on Yin in the body. It is the lowest area of the lower Dan Tian and can influence this entire Dan Tian. In qi gong this area is squeezed to stimulate its energetic properties and strengthen the local muscles. Squeezing this area also influences the top of the head. This acupoint is used in Yin–Yang treatments. Bai Hui, Du 20, is at the vertex. Both points have Hui in their name and stimulating one of them stimulates the other. Du 20 is often used to treat hemorrhoids. It is important to realize this area is connected to the Kidneys and influences Jing. The Chong, Ren, and Du channels meet at this point and Ren 1 can influence all three channels. Hui Yin is part of the marrow matrix that extends from the Kidneys to the umbilicus, to Hui Yin, and back to the Kidneys.

TREATMENT

Hui Yin influences the entire lower Jiao. It can treat conditions that manifest there, including damp, phlegm, blood stagnation, heat, and any combinations of them.

Ren 2   Qu Gu   Curved Bone

DESCRIPTION

Curved Bone is the pubic bone. The name is based on the point location.

TREATMENT

Regulates the lower Jiao, especially the Bladder and urination. Influences Jing, it is located near bone. It can guide Jing into bone. It benefits the Kidneys and essence.

Ren 3   Zhong Ji   Middle Pole   Central Pole

Bladder *mu*. The meeting of the three-leg Yin channels: Liver, Kidney, and Spleen.

DESCRIPTION

Zhong Ji is the name of the North Star, the center of the sky. The point is the center of the vertical and horizontal axis of the body. This point balances and centers a person.

TREATMENT

Treats any urination or Bladder problem, damp heat, enuresis, uterine bleeding, frequent urination, urinary tract infection, nocturnal emission, menstrual disorders, and tonifies the Kidneys.

Ren 4   Guan Yuan   Gate to the Original Qi   Origin Pass

Small Intestine *mu*. Meeting of the three-leg Yin channels.

DESCRIPTION

This is the location of the uterus (blood chamber), cinnabar field (Dan Tian) and life gate Fire (Ming Men). The area around this point is where Ming Men/the Gate of Vitality cooks Jing, creating source qi. Needling this point stimulates the production of source qi, and Kidney Yin and Kidney Yang.

TREATMENT

Nourishes or tonifies Yang, qi, Yin, and blood of the entire body. Tonifies the Kidneys. Regulates the uterus. Calms *shen*. Roots the *hun*. One of the best tonification points for the entire body.

Treats enuresis, nocturnal emission, frequent urination, irregular menses, uterine bleeding, postpartum hemorrhage, prolapse of rectum, infertility, fatigue, and dampness.

Ren 5   Shi Men   Stone Door   Stone Gate

San Jiao *mu*.

DESCRIPTION

Stone Gate can mean a blockage. It can be a blockage that prevents our ability to transform Jing to qi, and transport this qi throughout the body to support *shen*. Treating this point with other points can dissolve blockages and allow transformations, from ancestral or early life influences, to postnatal influences. This progression is necessary for growth and self-realization.

TREATMENT

Transforms and drains fluids throughout the body. Opens Water passages. Promotes urination. Treats diarrhea. Strengthens the original/Yuan qi and the Kidneys. Regulates the uterus. (Contraindicated for young females.) Treats edema, masses in the lower abdomen, nodules. The nodules can be from phlegm and blood accumulation.

Ren 6   Qi Hai   Sea of Qi

DESCRIPTION

Qi Hai influences the area that is a reservoir of qi for the entire body. Its location is the Dan Tian (qi field). It influences the lower Dan Tian in a similar way to Guan Yuan, Ren 4. The point influences the Kidneys and Jing, and prenatal substances. Qi Hai has a powerful ability to move qi; to move stagnations and patterns deep in the body. Qi Hai is a common location to focus attention in meditation. It grounds, roots, and centers. It relates to Jing, in the *shen–qi–Jing* model.

TREATMENT

Regulates qi and blood in lower Jiao. Tonifies qi and Yang. Tonifies Kidney qi, pre-Heaven, and Yuan qi.

Treats fatigue, abdominal pain, damp and hernia, genital disorders, enuresis, edema, asthma, diarrhea, dysentery, uterine bleeding, nocturnal emissions, and constipation.

Ren 8   Shen Que   Spirit Gate

DESCRIPTION

Que is a symbol for an empty space. This space functions to nourish the fetus. It also nourishes the Gate of Vitality and Jing, and the process of creating source qi. It has similar functions to Guan Yuan and Qi Hai. In Nei Dan, our awareness or consciousness moves through transformation and change that mirrors the *shen–qi–Jing* model. Shen Que assists in the transformation of Jing to qi, from ancestral to postnatal. Awareness transforms as Jing transforms to qi.

TREATMENT

Nourishes the fetus. Rescues and raises Yang, tonifies original qi. Tonifies Yang and the Spleen. Warms original Yang. Moves gastrointestinal qi, cock's crow diarrhea, borborygmus, and abdominal pain. This point is contraindicated for acupuncture; use moxibustion.

Ren 9   Shui Fen   Water Separation   Water Divide

DESCRIPTION

Shui Fen is located over the Small Intestine, which separates the pure from the impure; the separation is on both physical and psychological levels. It influences the Small Intestine's separation function. Along with other channels and points, Shui Fen can assist in the function of separating issues, situations, and conditions in life. When we cannot see with clarity and distinguish situations, consider this point in the treatment. The Small Intestine allows us to see with clarity and separate, the Gallbladder allows for selection among choices, and the Kidneys provide the willpower to take action and implement the choice.

TREATMENT

Promotes the transformation of fluids and controls Water passages. It transforms damp, phlegm, and edema of the whole body. Treats retention of urine, diarrhea, and ascites.

Ren 10   Xia Wan   Lower Epigastrium   Lower Controller

DESCRIPTION

The Lower Controller permits release of what is no longer necessary, which allows for new experiences. A balanced *yi* and the energetics of the Stomach and Spleen hold and release. The Spleen holds blood in the vessels and it also holds emotions. Xia Wan allows the releasing of experiences and emotions the *yi* holds. Xia Wan assists in releasing emotions.

TREATMENT

Promotes the descending of Stomach qi. Relieves stagnation of food. Treats the lower part of the Stomach (pylorus). Tonifies the Spleen.

Ren 11   Jian Li   Interior Strengthening

DESCRIPTION

Jian Li promotes a smooth flow in the middle Jiao, including the Spleen and Stomach. It also promotes smooth flow in changes in life, particularly related to the *yi* and thoughts and attachments. This point combined with other points can regulate the flow of thoughts that bring order, fluidity and harmony.

TREATMENT

Harmonizes and strengthens the middle Jiao. Descends Stomach qi. It treats vomiting, edema, and digestive conditions.

Ren 12   Zhong Wan   Middle of Epigastrium
Middle Controller

Stomach front *mu*. Influential point of the Fu organs. The meeting of the Small Intestine, San Jiao, and Stomach channels. Group luo point of the middle Jiao.

DESCRIPTION

The point is located in the middle of the abdomen and is the *mu* of the Stomach, the Earth element, and the center. This is the group luo of the middle Jiao. It influences the entire middle Jiao and all its functions, including the production of Gu qi. It assists in sending Gu qi to the Lungs to create Zhong qi. The Lung internal pathway originates in this location, and is the parent element of the Lungs. It has a strong influence on the Lungs. The point treats the *yi* spirit, which includes over-thinking, obsessive behavior, repetitive thinking, and worry. When moving to the center we are in the present moment, not the past or future, and this brings calmness and centeredness. Zhong Wan assists in digesting and transforming life experiences, keeping what is valuable, and letting go of what is not necessary. Zhong Wan relates to postnatal influences, especially imbalances related to our lifestyle and our choices in life. This point can assist in releasing from those imbalances, allowing a balanced condition as we move to the Heart center.

TREATMENT

Tonifies the Stomach and Spleen. Tonifies all Fu organs. Tonifies the Lungs. Treats all digestive conditions. Resolves damp and phlegm. Regulates qi in the middle Jiao. Treats insomnia due to excess in the Stomach. Treats dysentery, intestinal gas, vomiting, indigestion, insomnia, jaundice.

Ren 13   Shang Wan   Upper Epigastrium   Upper Controller

Meeting of the Stomach and Small Intestine channels. The point is located at the upper opening of the Stomach.

DESCRIPTION

Shang Wan is the Upper Controller and connects to the celestial. When this point is open and free flowing we are able to take in life experiences and digest them in a healthy and balanced way. If Shang Wan is open and functioning properly we move smoothly to Ju Que, the front *mu* of the Heart.

TREATMENT

Treats nausea, vomiting, hiccups, belching, Stomach pain. Subdues rebellious Stomach qi. Treats the fundus.

Ren 14   Ju Que   Great Palace   Great Tower Gate

Heart front *mu.*

DESCRIPTION

The point name has to do with its physical location. The breastbone looks like a gate to the commanding organ: the Heart. The point is the front *mu* of the Heart. The name "Great Tower Gate" reflects the front *mu* point as an entry to the Heart. Que can mean "a palace" and "empty space." This point is an entry to the Heart *shen* and treats Heart conditions, especially emotional conditions. When we feel empty, treating this point connects us to our Heart *shen*. It is the gate to our *shen*.

TREATMENT

Treats phlegm misting the Heart. Clears Heart heat. Regulates Heart qi. Stabilizes the spirit. Treats pain in the Heart and the chest. Treats mental disorders; calms the mind. Subdues rebellious Stomach qi. Treats difficulty swallowing. Regulates stagnations in the chest, palpitations, nausea.

Ren 15   Jiu Wei   Dove Tail

Luo point of the Ren channel. Source point of all Yin organs.

DESCRIPTION

The point name is related to the physical appearance and structure of the xiphoid process. A dove is a bird of love and peace. This point provides Yin, a nurturing and nourishing substance. If someone is lacking support or nourishment, consider Jiu Wei. If the treatment plan is to assist a person in enhancing bonding in their life, consider this point.

TREATMENT

Calms the *shen*, nourishes and benefits Yin of all organs, opens the chest.

Ren 16   Zhong Ting   Center Courtyard

DESCRIPTION

Zhong means the center and the Ren is the Sea of Yin. This point accesses the center of Yin to bring nourishment and support to the "courtyard," the *shen*. It can calm and center a person in their courtyard.

TREATMENT

Regulates accumulations in the chest.

Ren 17   Tan Zhong   Middle of Chest   Alchemical Altar Upper Sea of Qi   Chest Center

Pericardium *mu*, influential point of qi, meeting of the Spleen, Kidney, Pericardium, Small Intestine, and San Jiao. Group luo of the upper Jiao.

The name is based on its location in the chest and being the *mu* of the Pericardium. The Pericardium is the protector of the Heart.

Description

Tan Zhong is the group point of the upper Jiao. It influences the entire upper Jiao, which includes the Lungs, Pericardium, and Heart. It also influences the Lung *po* and the Heart *shen*, and their corresponding qualities and functions. From a Nei Dan perspective, this area influences the collective consciousness and conditioning of society. By cultivating this area we free ourselves from these influences, allowing awareness of our Yuan Shen.

Treatment

Tonifies and regulates the Lungs and Heart. It is important for qi development and assists the Heart to pump blood. Tonifies Zhong qi. Facilitates the dispersing and descending functions of the Lungs. Releases emotions related to the Heart. Treats Lung heat, palpitations, hiccups, asthma, chest pain, difficulty swallowing, resolves phlegm in the upper Jiao. Treats insufficient lactation.

Ren 18   Yu Tang   Jade Hall

Description

Jade is something precious, and a hall where it is located (Yu Tang) is a space where we can connect to wisdom within. This point is level with the Liver front *shu* point.

Treatment

Calms the *shen*. Regulates stagnations in the chest.

Ren 19   Zi Gong   *Purple Palace*

DESCRIPTION

Zi Gong is the "palace" of knowledge of the past, including our ancestors. This point can provide insight to our life. Zi Gong is level with the Heart front *shu*. It accesses wisdom and insight within our spirit.

TREATMENT

Calms the *shen*. Regulates stagnations in the chest.

Ren 20   Hua Gai   *Florid Canopy*

Hua Gai can mean the opening of a flower. This point is level with the Lung front *shu* point and the *po*. The *po* represents the physical body and its desires and pleasures.

DESCRIPTION

This point connects the *shen* with the *po*, allowing the blooming of our *shen* in our body.

TREATMENT

Treats local stagnations.

Ren 21   Xuan Ji   *Jade Pivot   Jade within the Pearl   North Star*

DESCRIPTION

Xuan Ji is a precious pivot that can align to heavenly treasures. The North Star is the center of the universe in Taoist cosmology and contains heavenly treasures. This point enables the treasures of life, contained in our spirit, to flow deep within.

TREATMENT

Treats local stagnations.

Ren 22   Tian Tu   Heavenly Prominence
Opening to the Heavens

Window of the sky point. Meeting of the Yin Wei channel.

DESCRIPTION

The windpipe is like a chimney of the upper Jiao and relates to Heaven in the cosmology of the body. The protrusion on either side of Tian Tu explains the alternative name, Celestial Protrusion. Tian Tu receives the heavenly treasures from the celestial, the head. Keeping this point and area open and flowing freely allows for a smooth flow and communication between Heaven and Humanity. It receives blood and qi from the neck and head, and allows us to express ourselves.

TREATMENT

Descends Lung qi, resolves phlegm and damp, clears heat, sudden hoarseness, difficult swallowing; facilitates and regulates movement of Lung qi, descends qi, and treats a sore and dry throat. Treats asthma, acute and chronic coughs, acute bronchitis, profuse sputum, goiter, and hiccups.

Ren 23   Lian Quan   Angular Ridge Spring

Meeting of the Yin Wei channel.

TREATMENT

Dispels interior wind, promotes speech, clears Fire, subdues qi, and resolves phlegm. Lian Quan can be used for speech conditions caused by wind-stroke.

Ren 24   Cheng Jiang   Sauce Receptacle

Ghost point. Meeting of the Du, Large Intestine, and Stomach channels.

DESCRIPTION

Chen Jiang can close the Ren channel to retain Yin. It can assist in nurturing the bonding process by keep the *yi* focused internally.

TREATMENT

Ren 24 has a strong influence on the face. It expels exterior wind and wind invading the face, and treats facial paralysis.

Confluent point (command, opening, master point)

- Lie Que, Broken Sequence, Lung 7.

- Luo point on the Lungs.

Coupled point

- Zhao Hao, Shining Sea, Kidney 6.

Other point qualities

- Jiu Wei, Dove Tail, Ren 15.

- Luo point. Connects to the Du channel.

- Source point of Yin organs.

Chapter 7

THE DU CHANNEL

Common names

- Governor channel
- Controlling channel
- Supervisor channel
- Sea of Individuality
- Sea of Separation
- Sea of Yang

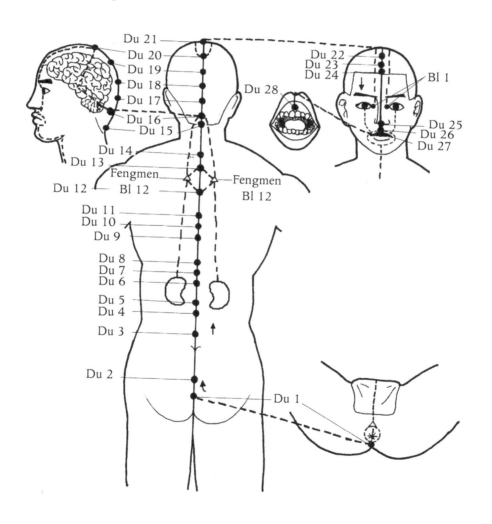

Figure 7.1 The Du channel

The Du channel is the Sea of Yang. Yang energetic properties include movement, activity, exploration, and independence. The energetic properties also include the natural expansion from the bonding and dependency that are characteristic during early life. This Yang expansion includes walking, talking, and interacting with new people and new locations, and having new experiences.

The independence and exploration process begins with energetic properties of Ming Men, the Gate of Vitality. This is a gate to qi, Yang, and Fire that ignites movement. If Ming Men or the moving qi between the Kidneys is deficient or suppressed, we might not move forward to interact with others. If we are held back, our Yang is suppressed and can lead to a lack of inspiration. It can prevent the Kidneys from grasping qi from the Lungs. This not grasping can be seen in our actions in life, and in not grasping life, not engaging in life. The vitality of Ming Men provides the willpower to allow the natural unfolding of exploration and interaction with other people, places, and activities.

Da Zhui, Du 14, is the meeting of Yang channels, and it influences Yang qi. This Yang qi allows us to stand upright, lift the head, and look outward to all around us. The area from Du 14 to Du 16 includes areas around the functions of voice and speech. Speech requires action. The Sea of Yang, or Du channel, has action as its fundamental function. The Du channel flows to the gums, mouth, and lips, to allow expression. As one explores new places, people, and experiences, the body has a built-in means of self-expression about them. Imbalances of the Du channel include the inability to express oneself. Du 15, Mute's Gate, can assist in treating this condition. Treating the Du channel can assist in releasing conditions preventing expression.

The Du channel desires to unite with the Ren channel. These two channels have internal pathways that connect to each other. As the Du unfolds, it always desires the comfort of the Ren channel and its bonding and synchronization. Du contains an innate intelligence to bring back to the Ren and the body its experiences, so they can be digested and processed. This processing allows us to mature, obtain wisdom, and develop the ability to make healthy choices. Having healthy interactions and processing leads to living a healthy, happy, and natural life. The ability to process obstructions and let go of what is not necessary, while retaining what is beneficial, is essential to living from our spirit.

As we experience, grow, and transform, our innate intelligence guides the Du to seek experiences that support our spirit. Our body, mind, and spirit become one integrated whole. The Du always likes to be able to explore and return to its root, which is the lower Jiao. The lower Jiao is the Yin area of the body and represents bonding, nurturing, and nourishment. The nourishing and bonding of the Ren needs to be unified with the exploration and independence of the Du. When harmonized, both qualities are expressed in our life. The Heavenly Orbit Nei Dan meditation helps harmonize the Yin and Yang, the Ren and Du channels.

Internal pathway

The Du channel originates in the lower abdomen and emerges from the perineum. It influences the lower Dan Tian, the genitals, and fertility.

It passes through Chiang Qiang, Du 1, and runs posteriorly along the midline of the sacrum, to the interior of the spinal column, to Feng Fu, Du 16, at the nape of the neck. It influences the lower Dan Tian, the spine, and the Kidneys.

It enters the Sea of Marrow, the brain. It influences the Jing-Shen, the brain.

It then ascends to the vertex at Bai Hui, Du 20, before descending along the midline of the head to the bridge of the nose and the philtrum at Du 26, Ren Zhong. The pathway terminates at the junction of the upper lip and gum. It influences the upper gums, lip, and the nose. The tongue connects the Ren and Du channels.

The Du channels internal pathway has three branches.

First branch

The pathway originates in the lower abdomen, descends to the genitals and the perineum, and winds around the anus. It then ascends inside the interior of the spinal column and enters the Kidneys. The Du channel sends Yang to stimulate the genitals. It can treat infertility and impotence.

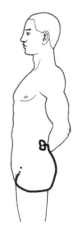

Second branch

The channel originates in the lower abdomen, winds around the external genitalia, and ascends to the middle of the umbilicus. It then passes through the Heart, ascends to the throat, winds around the mouth, and ascends to below the middle of the eyes. This branch connects to the Ren channel.

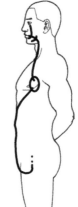

Third branch

The pathway emerges at Jing Ming, Bladder 1. It flows to the Bladder channel bilaterally along the forehead and converges at the vertex and enters the brain.

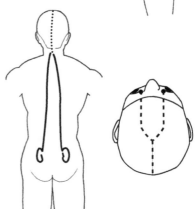

The pathway emerges at Feng Fu, Du 16, and then divides into two and descends through Feng Men, Bladder 12, along both sides of the spine, to the Kidneys. Some view the Hua Tua Jia Ji points as part of this pathway.

The Du pathway according to the Pulse Classic

Originates at the point of the lower extremity, Hui Yin, Ren 1, and joins the inside of the spine, reaching Feng Fu, Wind Mansion, Du 16, through the back.

Anatomical areas of influence

Anus, genitalia, back, spine, occiput, head, brain, and marrow. Controls Yang: qi, Yuan qi, Wei qi, heat, wind, Fire, activity, and movement.

Common conditions the Du channel treats

Pain and stiffness of the spine, pain in the eyes, headache, epilepsy, convulsions, opisthotonos, external wind, and cold attack. Influences Kidneys, Yang and qi, Spleen Yang deficiency. Circulates Wei qi, regulates heat, infertility, constipation, colic, hemorrhoids, enuresis, and influences the central nervous system.

Du channel points and functions

Du 1   Chiang Qiang   Long Strong   Lasting Strength

Luo point of the Du channel. Meeting point of the Ren, Gallbladder, and Kidney channels.

DESCRIPTION

The Du is the Sea of Yang, which is both long and strong. The first point on the channel is the beginning and influences the entire channel. The Du includes the spine, a long bone. Du 1 influences the entire channel and the skeletal system, making it long and strong.

TREATMENT

Regulates and opens the Ren and Du channels. Courses and regulates local channel qi. Treats damp heat in the lower Jiao. Calms the mind (bottom treating top, Yin treating Yang). Tonifies and strengths the anus muscle. Treats hemorrhoids, rectum prolapse, bloody stools and influences the spine and brain.

Du 2   Yao Shu   Lumbar Shu

Transporting point of the lumbar region.

DESCRIPTION

Yao Shu has a direct relationship to the Gate of Vitality and our life force. This life force is the root of our body, and is part of the lower Dan Tian. Flowing into this area is essential for qi to flow up the Du channel to the brain. The energetics of this point influence the eight sacral foramen points, where the spinal nerves flow through. Yao Shu influences the powerful energies flowing in the coccyx and sacrum.

TREATMENT

Extinguishes interior wind, pain, and stiffness of the lower back, and strengthens the lower back. Tonifies Kidney Yang and moves qi. Arouses Ming Men Fire. Treats epilepsy, calms spasms and convulsions. Used to treat hemorrhoids.

Du 3   Yao Yang Guan   Lumbar Yang Gate

Yao Yang Guan is a bridge from Hui Yin, Ren 1, to Ming Men, Du 4.

DESCRIPTION

This point stimulates the activity of moving qi to Ming Men, stimulating the essential function of the Gate of Vitality.

TREATMENT

Strengthens the lower limbs, lumbar region, and the lower back. Tonifies the Kidneys and expels cold damp.

Du 4   Ming Men   Gate of Life   Door of Life
Jing Gong   Palace of Essence

DESCRIPTION

The Door of Life is also called the Jade Capital and influences the Cinnabar Field. "Jade" means something precious, and the "Cinnabar Field" is a metaphor for the Dan Tian and the transformations that occur there. The Chinese believe life essence is between the Kidneys and behind and below the navel. This point accesses this area. Ming Men is the residence of essence. "Ming" can mean destiny. This point influences the *zhi* and the will to pursue and live the life you desire. It holds the willpower to fulfill your quest and destiny.

Treatment

Tonifies Kidney Yang and the gate of vitality. Tonifies source qi and essence. Reinforces the Kidneys. Warms and expels cold. Benefits the spine, back, knees, bone, and lower back. Treats infertility due to essence or Yang deficiency. Treats lumbago, impotence, irregular menses, diarrhea, leucorrhoea, and nocturnal emission.

Du 5   Xuan Shu   Suspended Axis

Description

Xuan Shu allows the energetics of Ming Men to continue in our life, to move up the ladder of our life (the Du channel and the 24 vertebra). This is the axis to continue in the transformation process.

Du 6   Ji Zhong   Spinal Center

Description

Ji Zhong is the center of the spine. The center is the place of balance and the space of change. This point assists in maintaining balance to support changes.

Treatment

Moves damp, tonifies the Spleen, and clears spinal heat. Regulates the spine.

Du 7   Zhong Shu   Central Axis

Description

Zhong Shu supports the action of change. When you want to begin change from a balanced state, this point can assist in new movements.

Treatment

Supports the digestive organs, harmonizes the Liver and Gallbladder, tonifies the Spleen, and moves damp.

Du 8   Jin Suo   Tendon Spasm   Sinew Contraction

Level with the Liver *shu*.

DESCRIPTION

Jin Suo supports flexibility in your life. Being flexible is essential in health and vitality.

TREATMENT

Relaxes the sinews, eliminates interior wind, soothes the Liver. Treats difficulty dealing with changes in life. Treats epilepsy, convulsions, muscle spasms, and gastric pain.

Du 9   Zhi Yang   Reaching Yang

Level with the seventh thoracic vertebra. Zhi means extreme, to reach.

DESCRIPTION

The point, which is on the Yang channel, is considered Yang within Yang. The upper body is Yang and Du 9 is below the seventh vertebra. Seven is an odd number and is Yang. (Odd numbers are Yang and even numbers are Yin.) Zhi Yang assists in enhancing Yang and qi, and moving a person into new directions and transformations. This point can stimulate qi to the brain, stimulating the Jing-Shen.

TREATMENT

Regulates the Liver and Gallbladder. Moves qi and opens the chest and diaphragm; treats hiccups, sighing. Relieves damp heat. Assists in bringing substances up the Du channel. It is used to treat jaundice.

Du 10   Ling Tai   Spirits Tower   Spirits Pagoda

DESCRIPTION

Reconnects a person to their spirit to continue their personal growth and transformation.

TREATMENT

Lung conditions. Local conditions.

Du 11   Shen Dao   Spirit Path

Level with the Heart *shu*. It is a path to one's spirit.

DESCRIPTION

This point assists in reconnecting to one's spirit. Some traditions use moxibustion, not acupuncture.

TREATMENT

Regulates the Heart. Treats palpitations, clears Heart Fire, quiets the Heart and spirit. Treats insomnia and calms the mind.

Du 12   Shen Zhu   Body Pillar   Spirit Pillar

Level with the Lung *shu*. Shen means "body, person." Zhu means "pillar, post, support." The point is between the shoulder blades and the third thoracic vertebra, and can be considered a pillar of the spine.

DESCRIPTION

This point reconnects us to the things that support us in our life. Shen Zhu influences Lung qi, which supports the body.

TREATMENT

Treats wind, calms spasms, tonifies Lung qi, strengthens the body, clears Lung and Heart heat. Treats the *po*. Use to treat cough, asthma, epilepsy.

Du 13   Tao Dao   Middle Path   Way of Happiness   Furnace of the Tao

Meeting of the Bladder channel.

DESCRIPTION

Assists in helping a person move through changes in life.

TREATMENT

Clears heat, expels wind, regulates Shao Yang. Use to treat alternating fever and chills.

Du 14   Da Zhui   Big Vertebra   Great Hammer

Meeting point of the six Yang channels. The Chinese call the vertebra "spine hammers." Da Zhui is the most prominent vertebra.

DESCRIPTION

Da Zhui connects the arms, legs, and head. When this area is open and flowing, it circulates qi throughout the body. This point assists in guiding qi into the Jing-Shen, the brain, and the crown (Bai Hui, Du 20).

TREATMENT

Clears Tai Yang, Shao Yang, and Yang Ming heat. Treats febrile disease, expels wind, releases the exterior, clears interior and exterior heat. Regulates Ying and Wei. Calms the *shen*. Tonifies Yang and Heart Yang. Stimulates the brain. Use to treat malaria, asthma, cough, and common cold.

Du 15   Ya Men   Mute's Gate

Window of the Sky, Nine Needles Return Yang, Yang Wei channel point.

DESCRIPTION

Mute's Gate assists a person to express themselves.

TREATMENT

This point connects to the root of the tongue and treats voice disorders. Clears the mind, stimulates speech, especially in children with speech problems; helps in post-stroke speech conditions. Clears the senses and restores consciousness. Extinguishes interior wind.

Du 16   *Feng Fu   Wind Palace   Wind Mansion*

Four-Sea of Marrow. Window of the Sky. Ghost point. Yang Wei point.

DESCRIPTION

The Du channel's internal pathway moves to the brain at this point. Wind can enter the body at this point/palace. Feng Fu can release pathogenic factors. It can also guide vital substances to and from this point and area of the body.

Wind can mean change. Our ability to respond to changes in life is essential to health and well-being. Feng Fu assists in adjusting and responding to change.

TREATMENT

Treats exterior and interior wind. Calms the *shen*. Benefits the brain and marrow. Used for wind-stroke, epilepsy, hemiplegia.

Du 17   *Nao Hu   Brain's Door*

Meeting of the Bladder channel.

DESCRIPTION

Nao Hu is a point that can guide a treatment into the brain, the Jing-Shen.

TREATMENT

Eliminates wind; benefits the eyes and brain; calms *shen* and spine pain.

Du 18   *Qiang Jian   Unyielding Spine*

This point is midway between Du 16 and Du 20.

DESCRIPTION

Du 16 and Du 20 have internal pathways to the brain. Located in the middle of them, Qiang Jian can influence both of the points and their ability to influence Yang. Qiang Jian can influence our will and determination to work through challenges, stagnations, and obstacles.

TREATMENT

Calms Yang and too much thinking.

Du 19   Hou Ding   Behind the Vertex

Hou Ding is behind Bai Hui, the vertex. Being behind, it can see clearly.

DESCRIPTION

This point assists in seeing influences in our life, especially from the past. These would include, for example, our family, ancestors, and society.

TREATMENT

Calms and soothes the spirit and mind. Can be used for intense emotional conditions. Local conditions.

Du 20   Bai Hui   Hundred Meetings   Hundred Convergences

Meeting point of all Yang channels. Alternate names are Five-fold Convergence, Linking Convergence, Mountain Top, Celestial Fullness, Mud Ball Palace.

DESCRIPTION

Bai Hui is a place of unity. It is the connection of Heaven and Earth, body and mind, and the physical and spiritual. There is an internal pathway from the Liver, which begins in the foot and flows to Bai Hui. This inner connection connects the feet, which are Earth, and the head, which is Heaven. Bai Hui allows integration of spiritual insights into the body. In some Nei Dan traditions, Bai Hui is place to make a connection to celestial energies and influences.

Raises Yang qi, especially Spleen qi. Strengthens the ascending function of the Spleen. Tonifies the Spleen. Calms or lifts the spirits and *shen*. Tonifies Yang. Pacifies wind. Assists in resuscitation. Benefits the brain. Sedates Yang. Treats headache. Clears the mind. Pacifies wind. Treats the vertex. Treats vertigo, coma, prolapse of the rectum, uterus, and Stomach, hemorrhoids. Assists in resuscitation, tinnitus, and dizziness. Use with caution if there is high blood pressure.

Du 21   Qiang Ding   Before the Vertex

DESCRIPTION

"Before" implies the prenatal. This point assists in understanding life before birth, and can offer insight to life after leaving this world. It can help when dealing with major transformations in life. Qiang Ding can assist in looking to the future.

TREATMENT

Calms the *shen*.

Du 22   Xin Hui   Fontanel Meeting

The cranial bones fuse here and the energy is sealed in.

DESCRIPTION

Xin Hui can assist in guiding qi and a treatment into the Jing-Shen, the brain, and the Yuan level. It can also help loosen up rigid, locked patterns.

TREATMENT

Brings qi to the head and the brain. Can be used as a guiding point to the brain.

Du 23   Shang Xing   Upper Star   Ming Tang
Hall of Brightness

In Taoist philosophy, humanity is a microcosm of Heaven, Humanity, and Earth. The head images the stars. Du 23 is at the front and top of the head; both are Yang.

DESCRIPTION

Shang Xing is a star close to the heavens and can provide guidance and direction. The Du channel has a strong connection to the brain and the Jing-Shen. This point influences the *shen* and emotions.

TREATMENT

Opens the nose. Treats epistaxis, rhinorrhea, and mostly chronic nasal problems.

Du 24   Shen Ting   Mind Courtyard   Spirit Court

Meeting of the Bladder and Stomach channels.

DESCRIPTION

The brain is considered the seat of the spirit, and the Du channel has pathways to the Heart *shen* and the brain, the Jing-Shen. Shen Ting influences both. This point calms the *shen*. When the *shen* is calm, we can gain insight and clarity.

TREATMENT

Calms emotions, especially chronic and intense conditions. Clears the mind. Clears mental disorders due to wind influencing the *shen*. Treats heat leading to mania.

Du 25   Su Liao   White Bone Hole

Raises Yang. Opens the orifices, the portals.

Du 26   Ren Zhong   Middle of Person

Ghost point, meeting of the Large Intestine and Stomach channels.

DESCRIPTION

The nose receives the five qi from Heaven, and the mouth receives the five flavors from Earth. Ren Zhong is between the two and relates to humanity. It unites Heaven and Earth. It is close to the junction of the Du and Ren channels, and connects the two. This is where Yin–Yang can separate, leading to unconsciousness. This point can unite Yin–Yang, leading to resuscitation.

TREATMENT

This is a classic point for acute and severe back pain, especially along the spine. Benefits the lumbar region and spine. Promotes resuscitation. Opens the orifices. Invigorates the entire Du channel. Stimulates the brain. Calms the spirit. Used to treat deviation of the mouth, epilepsy, coma, trismus, hysteria.

Du 27   Dui Duan   Extremity of the Mouth
Clears heat. Cold sores. Local conditions.

Du 28   Yin Jiao   Gum Intersection
Meeting of the Ren and Stomach channels. Treats local conditions.

Confluent point (command, opening, master point)

- Hou Xi, Back Ravine, Small Intestine 3.

Coupled point

- Shen Mai, Ninth Branch, Bladder 62.

Luo point

- Chang Qiang, Long Strong, Du 1.

Chapter 8

THE TWO WEI CHANNELS

Common names

- Yin Linking channels
- Yang Linking channels

The Wei channels are the linking channels. They link to Yin and Yang. The history of the Wei channels is very interesting. Their pathways and points are not described in the *Su Wen, Ling Shu,* or the *Nan Ching*. These classic texts say the following about the Wei channels: "Yang Wei is where all Yang meet and the Yin Wei is where all Yin meet." Based on these classic books, it would not be possible to find points to needle on the Wei channels.

The *Classic of Acupuncture and Moxibustion (Jia Yi Jing)*, 280 AD, presents the points on the Wei channels in Book III, the section on the primary channels. The information is presented along with their standard primary channel point qualities. (It is an interesting variance with Book II, Chapter 2, which presents the Eight Extraordinary Channels and contains the information found in the *Su Wen* and *Ling Shu*.) We do not have any original versions of this classic text, it was restored at a later time; it is believed a section on the points in the primary channels was added at a later date. It is not until around the Ming dynasty that the Wei channels pathways are fully described with their points.

Wei channels allow access to the energetic properties of Yang and Yin in the body. They provide a framework to evaluate conditions of the three ancestries. Wei channels' energetic properties can access experiences as we age: the experiences that have caused imbalances within a person. These imbalances relate to significant stages in our life—for example, going to school for the first time, going through adolescence, career, marriage, menopause, etc. The imbalances include our responses to events and our activities as we travel through cycles of seven and eight years. Problems during these transitional periods can be diagnosed with Wei channel theory and treated with these channels.

Wei channels access issues of the past and future, their patterns and imprints. Are you living in the past? If you are, it is a Yin Wei issue. Are you always thinking of the future? If you are, it is a Yang Wei issue. Being trapped in time, past or future, relates to the Wei channels. It takes qi, blood, and, over the long term, Jing, to maintain this state of being "caught in time." It is very draining to maintain these conditions.

Structure is Yin and activities are Yang. Yin Wei energetic properties include how we respond to changes in our Yin over time. Yin includes our body shape, form, and appearance. It is our response to changes in Yin that can create imbalances. This includes how we feel about the way we look physically. If there are difficulties in this area, consider treating the Yin Wei channel.

Yang Wei reflects our activities, actions, and movements. If we have difficulties with what we do and how we do it, including our work, consider treating the Yang Wei channel.

Wei channels reflect our relationship with time. Are you living in past events, past relationships, or past professions? Are you always thinking of what you might be, what you will do, instead of living in the present time? If a desire to be something else or someone else is very strong, it can create a polarity that is at our deepest core. The polarity can vary in intensity. If it is very deep, it can cause profound disturbances. Understanding this dynamic allows the practitioner to design treatment plans to release this attachment to the past or future, using the Wei channels. As a treatment strategy, the practitioner can select channels and points that redirect or guide a person's *yi* or focus to their *shen*. For example, after treating the Wei channels, select Ling Dao, Spirit Pathway, Heart 4. Ling Dao can guide someone's focus on their spirit, providing insight and inspiration to live from their spirit, not the imbalances. Other channels and points can be used along with Ling Dao. When we use the full range of channels and points, we follow the tradition of the *Ling Shu*, the *Spiritual Compass*.

Points on the Wei channels can assist in moving us past stagnations from the past or future. There are cleft points on these channels, which indicate the channel is very susceptible to stagnations. These channels and points can access and treat stagnations. A classic symptom of the Yin Wei is Heart pain. This is a Yin Wei condition. The pain is not always physical pain. It can be emotional. Wei channel energetic properties allow us to determine whether the imbalance stems from the past, or desires of the future, and provides channels and points to treat the conditions.

The Yang Wei is comprised mostly of Tai Yang, Shao Yang, and Du channel points. The most points are from the Shao Yang/Gallbladder channel. The Gallbladder is a unique organ and channel. It is a Fu and Extraordinary organ. It is closely related to the Eight Extraordinary Channels and the Fu organs, and a bridge between the two. As a Shao Yang channel, it is a bridge or hinge between the inside and outside. From a Yang Wei perspective, it is the hinge between the external experiences in life and how we process them internally. Its ability to filter what is valuable and retain it, and release what is not valuable, is crucial to health. Both of the Wei channels can be used to access imbalances and let go of them, which would include a reducing needling method. They can also be reinforced to guide vital substances to the channels, points, and energy centers. This dynamic also works on the five *shen*, especially the *yi*. A reducing treatment can release one's mind, *yi*, or attention, away from the imbalance. A reinforcing method can guide one's focus or *yi* into channels, organs, or energy centers.

As we interact with people and life, the Yang Wei takes our experiences into the body and brain (Jing-Shen). The Yang Wei pathway goes into the Window of the Sky points: Yao Men, Du 15, Feng Fu, Du 16, and to the brain. The pathway includes the Tai Yang and Du channels. These channels include Yang energetic properties and are about activity, extending outward and experiencing life. Yang Wei includes how we process these experiences. If there is resistance or difficulty in processing the experiences, imbalances can occur. The Wei channels reveal the way the body filters: the way we take in, digest, and retain experiences and emotions is reflected in the signs and symptoms of that process. Classic symptoms include alternating fever and chills; this is when something is caught or stuck in the middle/Shao Yang, and cannot be processed properly. Shao Yang is a pivot point for processing. The Yang Wei can help people move out of stagnations, particularly during significant stages of life and human development.

Li Shi-Zhen believed the three-leg channels meet at Jin Men, Bladder 63. To him it was a Yang meeting point. This is one reason why it was selected to be on the Yang Wei pathway. Li Shi-Zhen adds Gallbladder 29 to the Wei channel; it is also on the Yang Qiao channel. Both channels also meet at Small Intestine 10. These two points are a major point combination to release those channels.

Chapter 9

THE YANG WEI CHANNEL

Common names
- Yang Linking channel
- Preserver of Yang
- Yang Tie Vessel
- Vessel of Yang Keeper

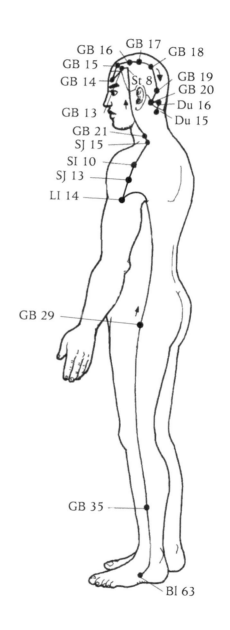

Figure 9.1 The Yang Wei channel

Internal pathway

The pathway originates near the heel at Jin Men, Bladder 63, at the junction of the foot Tai Yang channel, and emerges at the external malleolus. It ascends along the external/lateral malleolus and the Gallbladder channel of the leg, to pass through the hip region. The pathway ascends along the postero-lateral costal region to the posterior axillary fold, by Nao Shu, Small Intestine 10. It then crosses the top of the shoulder at Tian Liao, San Jiao 15, and Jian Jing, Gallbladder 21, and ascends along the neck to the ear and the forehead at Ben Shen, Gallbladder 13. The pathway crosses the head through the points of the Gallbladder channel as far as Feng Chi, Gallbladder 20, and then connects with the Du channel at Feng Fu, Du 16, and Ya Men, Du 15.

The channel flow follows the following channels: Tai Yang, Shao Yang, Tai Yang, Shao Yang, Du channels.

The Yang Wei pathway according to the Pulse Classic

The Yang Linking channel originates at the meeting of the various Yang and links all Yang.

Anatomical areas of influence

The channel influences the lateral aspect of the legs, hips, back, head, ears, and brain. It includes the Shao Yang temporal areas.

Common conditions the Yang Wei channel treats

Connects or links all Yang channels; dominates the exterior of the body, exterior syndromes such as chills and fever; conditions of the sides of the body, especially the shoulders and hips; ear conditions, vertigo, headache; muscle fatigue, pain, and distension in the waist; and Shao Yang conditions.

Yang Wei channel points and functions

Bladder 63   Jin Men   Metal Gate
Bladder cleft.

DESCRIPTION

Jin Men is the origin of the Yang Wei channel pathway. It deals with Lung and Metal issues that influence the exterior. The Lungs control the exterior. They open to the nose and have a strong relationship to the environment. Metal qi flows inward in the Five Phases. The energetic properties of the point are turning experiences into the body. Men is an exterior structure, an entrance or exit. Metal is the parent of Water and there is a giving relationship to Water. Metal, the Lungs, and the *po* bring life experiences deeper into the body to be processed and organized. This process contributes to our personality and constitution. This point can guide the processing of experiences deep in the body, or release unfavorable attachments or aspects of our life.

The Du channel represents the aspect of our self that explores the world and brings experiences into the body; the Yang Wei channel and its energetic properties assist in that process. The Yang Wei channel influences the experiences we are attached to and cannot let go. Treating Jin Men can begin the process of releasing our attachment to them.

TREATMENT

Clears blockages and stagnations. Calms *shen*. Moves one when stuck in cycles of time. Opens the orifices. It treats pain along the channel. Enhances the ability to process our experiences of life. Releases attachments, patterns, and conditioning.

Gallbladder 35   Yang Jiao   Yang Intersection
Yang Convergence

Yang Wei cleft point.

DESCRIPTION

The energetic properties of this point helps move one past blockages and stagnations. It is a junction of Yang and can influence Yang correspondences. The correspondences include thoughts, movement, activity, and actions. This point, along with other points in a treatment, can release one from the intensity of Yang correspondences of the Yang Wei. As a Yang junction, it can also assist in gathering and directing Yang into the body or releasing it.

Yang Wei cleft points are on the legs and deal with movement and the stagnations that may result from imbalances in movement. They can include too much movement or activity; they can also include lack of movement in life. Cleft points influence difficulties with Shao Yang energetic properties, the relationship between the outer and inner. They assist in allowing us to move through this tension of processing or filtering between the exterior and interior. Smooth processing or flowing allows for the free flow in our life.

TREATMENT

Invigorates, clears, and moves the channel. Stops pain. Calms *shen*. Yang comes together here. The three-leg Yang channels meet here. Gathers or releases Yang.

Gallbladder 29   Ju Liao   Squatting Bone Hole

This is a major release point for the Yang Wei and Yang Qiao channels. Both channels meet at Ju Liao, and it can release both channels.

DESCRIPTION

Ju Liao is located at the hip bone. Bones are part of the marrow matrix: Jing, marrow, bones, and the brain. Imbalances can enter this bone hole and enter into the marrow level. It can access and release old patterns and imbalances.

TREATMENT

Combined with other points on the Yang Wei and other channels, it can release imbalances throughout the body.

Small Intestine 10   Nao Shu   Upper Arm Shu

Nao Shu assists in bringing out pathogens locally and throughout the body. The upper arm allows movement of the upper limb; Ju Liao, Gallbladder 29, assists in moving the lower limb. Combining these two points releases the Yang Wei and Yang Qiao channels and their energetic properties. Nao Shu is a major release point.

Large Intestine 14   Bi Nao   Upper Arm

Removes local obstructions.

San Jiao 13   Nao Hui   Upper Arm Convergence

Regulates Shao Yang. Clears internal heat.

San Jiao 15   Tian Liao   Heavenly Crevice

The Yang Qiao and Gallbladder channels meet here.

DESCRIPTION

Tian Liao connects Heaven and Earth, qi and bones, *shen* and Jing. This crevice is a space to receive celestial guidance and draw it into the bone and Jing level. Things can get stored here, and can be released from this point. Shao Yang is a hinge and filtering process. When the Shao Yang process is functioning well it can retain what is necessary and release what is not.

Gallbladder 21   Jian Jing   Shoulder Well

DESCRIPTION

The shoulders contain the power to carry on with the work of life. Jian Jing connects to some of the most powerful points on the body, the Jing Well points. These points treat any organ and channel condition, and stimulate the qi of the channel. Jian Jing is a way to stimulate these points to stimulate the body. The other points in the treatment guide the qi to the organs, channels, and areas to be treated.

TREATMENT

Opens the Jing Well points. This is a major release point for the local muscular and channel systems. It has a powerful downward influence.

Gallbladder 13   Ben Shen   Mind Root   Spirit Root

DESCRIPTION

Ben Shen means "spirit root." The Gallbladder and Liver are Yin–Yang pairs and are the Wood element. These two Wood channels connect the feet, which are Earth, and the head, which is Heaven. The Liver has an internal pathway to the vertex and influences the brain and the *shen*. The Gallbladder channel flows around the temporal and occipital areas, influencing the brain and the *shen*.

The Gallbladder is both a Fu organ and a Curious organ. The translation for "Curious organs" could have been "Extraordinary organs." There is a strong connection between the Gallbladder and the Eight Extraordinary Channels. The Kidneys have the most points on the Eight Extraordinary Channels, and the Gallbladder has the second most points. The Gallbladder channel has a strong influence on the brain/Jing-Shen.

TREATMENT

Ben Shen can access the root of an emotional or spiritual condition. Calms the *shen*. Gathers essence and vital substances to the Sea of Marrow, the brain. Clears the brain. Increases willpower. By connecting to the root of our spirit, it can be a source of inspiration by gaining insight to our original nature.

Gallbladder 14   *Yang Bai   Yang White*

Brings brightness to your life, especially to the Lung *po*. Yang Bai assists in the connection of Heaven and the *po*.

Gallbladder 15   *Tou Lin Qi   Falling Tears*
Head Overlooking Tears

DESCRIPTION

Tou Lin Qi can assist in releasing imbalances from the Liver and the Gallbladder from the eyes. The Liver and Gallbladder channels open to the eyes and correspond to the *hun* spirit. The Gallbladder channel begins at the outer canthus and is a location to release imbalances from the *hun*.

TREATMENT

Calms the *shen*. Balances emotions. Yang Wei releases can come out of the eyes in the form of tears (similar to Foot Overlooking Tears, Gallbladder 41). Brightens the eyes.

Gallbladder 16   *Mu Chuang   Window of Eye*

DESCRIPTION

The Gallbladder and Liver correspond to the *hun* spirit, which reflects the collective nature of life. Mu Chuang can assist in helping a person perceive the unity of all people and all of life. Mu Chuang assists in connecting to the deep unity and wisdom from our inner eyes, the *hun* spirit, and the inseparable nature of all of life.

TREATMENT

Benefits the eyes. Expels wind. Subdues Liver yang. Increases insight.

Gallbladder 17   Zheng Ying   Upright Construction
Correct Plan

Description

Zheng Ying assists in the Gallbladder's ability to be decisive in decision-making. Based on the insights of the Liver *hun*, the energetic properties of this point allow us to follow a correct and good plan.

Treatment

Subdues Liver Yang. Calms the spirit.

Gallbladder 18   Cheng Ling   Spirit Receiver   Spirit Support

Description

Cheng Ling is the receiver of Heaven's vibrations. Spirit language includes vibration and frequency. In qi gong and Nei Dan, the chin is tucked in gently, aligning the crown and Cheng Ling to attune to celestial energies. The Shao Yang channel is the filter, the qi field connecting the inner and outer. It is a receiver of spiritual insights. It is a conduit of insight.

Treatment

Calms *shen*. Increases vitality or zest for life.

Gallbladder 19   Nao Kong   Brain Hollow
Vastness of the Brain

Description

Nao Kong is a portal to Jing-Shen, the brain, and a means to guide a treatment into the Jing-Shen. It is a way to attune to the unlimited nature of our life.

The ancients perceived the relationship between Jing and *shen*. They understood that each influenced the other. Our actions in life become our constitution and lodge in our Jing. The patterns and imprints in our Jing can block our connection to our *shen*. If we do not cultivate ourselves, we live from our patterns. Nei Dan or spiritual cultivation clears the patterns and blockages, revealing our spirit. With practice we become a living expression of our spirit. Our spirit infuses into Jing.

TREATMENT

Helps empty the brain. Clears the mind. Guides the treatment to the Sea of Marrow, the brain.

Gallbladder 20   Feng Chi   Wind Pond

DESCRIPTION

Wind can mean change. The classic books *Su Wen*, *Ling Shu*, and *I Ching* present change as a fundamental aspect of life. It is essential to understand change to understand health, harmony, and longevity. The first chapter in the *Su Wen* presents cycles of seven and eight years that humans move through, and Chapter 2 includes the four seasons. Understanding change and how to live in harmony with it is the basis of Chinese philosophy and medicine.

The Gallbladder channel is the Wood element, which corresponds to wind and change. When we are rigid, locked, and stagnant, we cannot respond effectively to changes in our environment and changes in our life. As a point on the Shao Yang channel, Gallbladder 20 can release pathogens that block and cause stagnation in the Shao Yang channel's energetic properties of turning, twisting, bending, adapting, adjusting, and responding. Feng Chi releases pathogens that prevent efficient interaction with change, allowing for healthy decision-making, decisive activity, and the smooth flow of movement in our daily life.

TREATMENT

Calms *shen*. Tonifies marrow. Nourishes the brain. Clears pathogenic wind. Helps one to adjust to deal with changes in life.

Du 15   Ya Men   Mute's Gate
Window to the Sky.

DESCRIPTION

"Mute's Gate" has a dual meaning. When we turn inward to connect to marrow or the Yuan level, there is no need to speak. Chinese philosophy is center-based. By turning inward to the center, we connect to our core and enter a deep peace and bliss. In this deep realization of our Yuan level, there is no need to speak. Ya Men has a pathway that flows to the brain. This pathway allows access to influence the brain (Jing-Shen).

Ya Men can also promote our ability to express ourselves verbally. Stimulating both the tongue and the brain, it can facilitate expression. Often the inability to communicate is the branch of a root condition. Treating the root should be included in the treatment.

TREATMENT

Clears the mind. Restores consciousness. Promotes the flow of Yang qi to the brain. Ya Men assists in verbal self-expression.

Du 16   Feng Fu   Wind Palace   Wind Mansion
Sea of Marrow. Window to the Sky. Ghost point.

DESCRIPTION

Feng Fu is a location to influence wind or change. The Du channel is the Sea of Yang, and wind is Yang. The head is Yang, compared to the feet, which are Yin. Feng Fu is an entry into the head and the brain. The brain is part of the marrow matrix and is susceptible to becoming rigid and stagnant. Feng Fu opens the flow of qi to the brain and crown, and then down the front of the body, following the Ren channel. This is the microcosmic orbit and a major aspect of Nei Dan.

TREATMENT

Feng Fu can release interior or exterior wind, and stimulates the brain. Calms the *shen*. Benefits the brain. Eliminates wind. Assists in dealing with change, wind, in one's life. Feng Fu assists in releasing old patterns in the marrow and the brain, allowing for a new way to respond to new experiences.

Confluent point (command, opening, master point)

- Wai Guan, Outer Gate, San Jiao 5.

Coupled point

- Zu Ling Qi, Foot Overlooking Tears, Gallbladder 41.

Cleft points

- Yang Jiao, Yang Intersection, Gallbladder 35, cleft of the Yang Wei channel.

- Ji Men, Metal Gate, Bladder 63, cleft of the Bladder channel.

Chapter 10

THE YIN WEI CHANNEL

Common names

- Yin Linking channel
- Yin Regulating channel
- Yin Tie channel
- Vessels of Aging

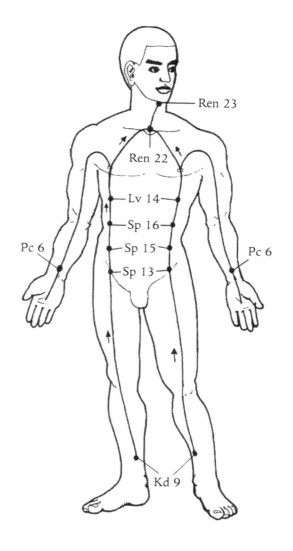

Figure 10.1 The Yin Wei channel

Internal pathway

The pathway originates at the medial aspect of the leg, Zhu Bin, Guest House, Kidney 9. It ascends along the medial aspect of the leg and thigh to the lower abdomen, to communicate with the Spleen channel at Fu She, Spleen 13; then Da Heng, Spleen 15, and Fu Ai, Spleen 16. It then runs along the chest, crossing the ribs at Qi Men, Liver 14, and ascends to the throat and neck. It meets the Ren channel at the neck, Tian Tu, Ren 22, and Lian Quan, Ren 23.

The pathway flows through the following channel: Shao Yin, Tai Yin, Jue Yin, Ren channels.

The Yin Wei pathway according to the Pulse Classic

Yin Linking channel originates at the confluence of the various Yin, and links all Yin.

The classics state that if Yin and blood are deficient, the Heart is not nourished, and this can lead to rib, chest and Heart pain, palpitations, and restlessness. We can use the Yin Wei to treat those conditions. The pathway goes to the chest and the head, and it includes the Kidney front *shu* points, which relate to the five Yin organs and the five *shen*.

Anatomical areas of influence

The channel influences Yin, blood, mental and emotional conditions, chest, Heart, Liver, *shen*, and the hypochondrium.

Common conditions the Yin Wei channel treats

Treats interior syndromes; moves and tonifies blood; treats chest pain (including chronic chest pain); controls the chest, Heart, and blood (cardiovascular system), fullness and pain of the lateral costal region; hypertension; upper abdomen; stomachache; lumbar pain. Tonifies Yin. Also treats psychological conditions: anxiety, fear, hysteria, nightmares, and depression.

Yin Wei channel points and functions

Kidney 9   Zhu Bin   Guest House

Yin Wei cleft point. When we are lost and disconnected from others and life, seeing a friend or friendly guest can bring awareness of our deep self, our *shen*—hence the name "Guest House."

DESCRIPTION

The Kidneys house our Jing and the *zhi* spirit, and are the Water element. Those qualities reflect the deepest, core aspect of our life. Zhu Bin allows us to see our own reflection, as if looking into a pool of Water. It enables us to look at ourselves in a non-judgmental way, to see ourselves clearly, not based on past experiences and conditions. When included in certain treatments, the influence of Zhu Bin can help a person exert willpower and realize their Yuan nature.

TREATMENT

Zhu Bin can treat emotional conditions from past experiences. It regulates and moves the Yin Wei channel. Treats Shao Yin conditions. Calms the *shen*. Treats phlegm misting the Heart, and opens the chest.

Spleen 13   Fu She   Bowel Abode

Fu She is a space to collect and store our connection to Earth, nourishment, and transformation.

DESCRIPTION

Fu She grounds us when the *yi* is too active and scattered. It allows one to hold things. It can assist in holding favorable aspects of the *yi*: your thoughts. It can also release the *yi* from repetitive and obsessive thoughts. It can move qi, both inward and outward.

Spleen 15   Da Heng   Great Horizontal

Da Heng is at the level of the umbilicus, the center of the body.

DESCRIPTION

Da Heng can ground and root someone in their center; the center is the root of our life. It can quiet the *yi*, allowing awareness of our *shen*. From the horizon we can see all the directions in our life, and so choose a clear path to move and interact. Da Heng can assist in releasing emotions and thoughts we have held onto for a long time. It assists in rooting the *yi* and calming the ego. It can tonify the Spleen and *yi*. It regulates the Large Intestine and Stomach. It can strengthen the limbs and assists in sending essence to the limbs.

Spleen 16   Fu Ai   Abdominal Lament

DESCRIPTION

The *yi* corresponds to our thoughts and thinking. It is the conceptual body that organizes our experiences, based on our life experience. Our accumulated life experiences create the way our *yi* filters and processes our experiences. When we suffer from overthinking, repetitive thinking, or unfavorable thoughts, they can trigger unfavorable emotions. Fu Ai can calm the *yi*. In this calmness and space, we can reconnect to our spirit and see the situation in a balanced way.

TREATMENT

Fu Ai calms and treats the *yi*, including repetitive and obsessive thoughts and behavior. When one is not properly nourished, Fu Ai assists in reducing unhealthy cravings. It can regulate the intestines.

Liver 14   Qi Men   Cycle Gate   Gateway of Hope

Liver *mu* point.

DESCRIPTION

The Liver is responsible for the smooth flow of qi and emotions. This flow includes lifelong cycles. Qi Men assists in resetting and attuning to the cycles of life. The Liver corresponds to the *hun,* the ethereal spirit and Jue Yin. The Liver is Wood, and its basic nature is to rise and flow upward. When a condition is very deep, in the Jue Yin stage it requires a force to move it up and out of the body. Qi Men can create a new cycle for a deep condition. It can help move a stagnant pattern. If you are stuck in past experiences, Qi Men can help release the attachment. The energetic properties of the Liver and Cycle Gate can profoundly move one past old, deep, Yuan level conditions. With a new cycle comes new hope for the future.

TREATMENT

Qi Men calms the *hun* and *yi* interactions, especially Wood overacting on Earth. It calms and roots the *hun.* Moves and tonifies blood. Promotes the smooth flow of Liver qi. It adjusts one to cycles of time and rhythms. It synchronizes.

Ren 22   Tian Tu   Heavenly Prominence
Opening to the Heavens

Window of the Sky point. Meeting of the Yin Wei channel.

DESCRIPTION

The windpipe is like a chimney of the upper Jiao and relates to Heaven in cosmology of the body. The protrusion on either side of Ren 22 explains the alternative name "Celestial Protrusion." Tian Tu receives the heavenly treasures from the celestial, the head. Keeping this point and area open and free flowing permits a smooth flow and communication between Heaven and Humanity.

TREATMENT

Descends Lung qi, resolves phlegm; clears damp, clears heat; treats sudden hoarseness, difficulty swallowing; facilitates and regulates movement of Lung qi, and dry throat. Used to treat asthma, acute and chronic cough, acute bronchitis, profuse sputum, goiter, and hiccups.

Ren 23   Lian Quan   Angular Ridge Spring (Adam's Apple)

DESCRIPTION

Lian Quan increases the ability to express oneself and communicate.

TREATMENT

Dispels interior wind, promotes speech, clears Fire, subdues qi, and resolves phlegm. Lian Quan is used for speech conditions resulting from wind-stroke.

Confluent point (command, opening, master point)

- Nei Guan, Inner Gate, Pericardium 6.

Coupled point

- Gong Sun, Yellow Emperor, Spleen 4.

Xi cleft point

- Zhu Bin, Guest House, Kidney 9.

Chapter 11

THE TWO QIAO CHANNELS

Common names

- Bridge channels
- Vessels of one's Stance
- Polarization of Yin–Yang
- Vessels holding pathologies

The Qiao channels are about structure. These channels have a close relationship to Wei qi and the sinew channels. A major aspect of the Qiao channels' energetic properties is that they deal with current conditions based on past or future influences. They represent the present-moment aspect of time.

The Qiao channels can release pathology from the past that is being experienced in the present. They can also release stresses about the future that are affecting the present moment. The stresses can influence our physical stance, structure, or posture. They can also influence our psycho-emotional stance, which can be our self-esteem.

Chapter 29 of the *Nan Jing* states: "The [two] Qiao channels are each an extension or reflection of the opposite state in the other: a disharmony in one causes the opposite disharmony in the other." This can be viewed as the mutual consumption theory of Yin–Yang.

Classical descriptions of the Yin Qiao include: Yin is tense and Yang is relaxed. When there are a lot of Yin qualities, there are fewer Yang qualities, and a person may have fatigue and want to sleep a lot. Also, with an accumulation of Yin, there can be abdominal heaviness, leucorrhoea, cold constriction, and cold pain.

For the Yang Qiao the opposite is the case: when Yang is tense, Yin is flaccid. Symptoms are insomnia, irritability, possible seizures, vertigo, and high fever.

The Qiao channels have pathways to the eyes, and include the way we look, our perception.

- Yin Qiao: How I look at myself. I am looking internally.

- Yang Qiao: How I look out to the external environment. I am looking out to the world.

The Kidneys and Bladder are Yin–Yang pairs, and they represent polar opposites. Emphasis on one of them diminishes the influence of the other. They influence each other. The confluent points for the Qiao channels are on the Kidney and Bladder channels. The Kidneys represent Yin. Yin includes the interior, and movement inward. The Bladder represents Yang. Yang includes the exterior, the outer world, and movement outward. Both Qiao channels go to Jing Ming, Bladder 1. They both influence the eyes, sleep, and how we see.

Chapter 26 of the *Nan Jing* identifies the Yang network vessel as the Yang Qiao, and the Yin network vessel as the Yin Qiao; the networks are the luo channels, which are containers that hold pathology. The *Nan Jing* is explaining the relationship between the luo and Qiao channels; if the luo channels are not cleared and released, they are deposited into the constitutional level, the Qiao channels. For example, trauma or chronic emotional stresses that are not resolved, and not let go, can be deposited in the Qiao channels.

Qiao channels harmonize Yin–Yang. They can also polarize each other. When one side is hyperactive, the other is hypoactive, to maintain a level of homeostasis in the body. This polarization can also create imbalances in the channels.

Qiao deals with current situations in life. Qiao channels harmonize or cope with current problems, current polarized situations. Imbalances can be on a physical level—for instance, gait, skeletal, bone, and postural conditions. Imbalances can include psycho-emotional conditions that relate to self-esteem, which may influence posture, structure, and skeletal conditions.

Yang Qiao

Yang Qiao channel energetic properties include your stance and actions in relationship to others. The Yang Qiao also supports the Du channel, in its Sea of Yang role of exploration. The Du and Yang Qiao have become popular coupled paired channels.

The Yang Qiao is activated when one is overly engaged with the exterior. The more intense the engagement, the more intense pathogens move to the exterior and activate imbalances in the Yang Qiao channel. When focus is at the exterior, your Wei qi is engaged at the exterior and you are not in the present moment, leading to exuberance of qi and possibly Yang rising, headaches, and hypertension. Directing your energy and desires too much towards others can lead to rebellious qi, which can cause rebellious actions—for example, nausea, headaches, and vomiting. When our thoughts, desires, and cravings are too active, it causes the body to be too active as well. It is the body following the mind. Slowing the mind down allows the body to slow down. This slowing down allows us to gain our stance and the opportunity to obtain balance.

Yin Qiao

Yin Qiao energetic properties include your stance in relation to yourself. The Yin Qiao reflects self-esteem. When we have self-esteem conditions, we may withdraw from interacting with other people. We can turn inward to escape from interacting with others. This situation can result from loss of a loved one, depression, or trauma; this is a polarization and a Yin Qiao condition. If you can't accept yourself in the current moment, or don't feel good about yourself, consider treating the Yin Qiao channels to release from this condition. The treatment should include additional channels and points that redirect a person to their spirit.

Chapter 12

THE YANG QIAO CHANNEL

Common names

- Yang Heel
- Yang Bridge
- Yang Motility
- Accelerator of Yang
- Yang Walker vessel
- Yang Stance channel

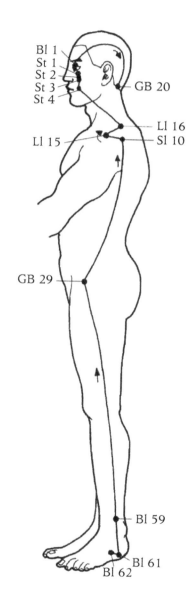

Figure 12.1 The Yang Qiao channel

Internal pathway

The channel originates at the lateral side of the heel at Shen Mai, Bladder 62, and flows to Pu Can, Bladder 61. It flows upward along the lateral malleolus and passes the posterior border of the fibula, Fu Yang, Bladder 59. The channel ascends to the lateral side of the thigh to the hip, Ju Liao, Gallbladder 29, and then goes along the posterior/lateral side of the hypochondrium to the posterior axillary fold. It then winds over the shoulder and ascends along the neck to the corner of the mouth. The pathway ascends to the cheek and alongside the nose to the inner canthus, Jing Ming, Bladder 1, to communicate with the Yin Qiao channel. It runs further upward along the Foot Tai Yang Bladder channel to the forehead. It then curves across the temporal region and descends to meet with Feng Chi, Gallbladder 20, and then enters the brain.

The Yang Qiao Pathway according to the Pulse Classic

The channel originates in the heel, it ascends to the lateral malleolus and submerges in the Wind Pool, Gallbladder 20.

Anatomical areas of influence

Lateral aspect of the legs, hips, back, neck, head, eye, and the brain.

Common conditions the Yang Qiao channel treats

Diseases of the eyes. Regulates the motion of the lower limb, eversion of the foot with tension and pain on the lateral aspect of the lower leg, and the medial side of the leg is flaccid, weak, or atrophied. Pain in the back and lumbar region, spasm of the lower limb, conditions of the lateral aspect of the body, hemiplegia, epilepsy, insomnia, redness and pain of the inner canthus. Includes conditions of excess Yang, especially in the head and neck, including cerebral thrombosis and hemorrhaging.

Yang Qiao channel points and functions

Bladder 62   Shen Mai   Ninth Channel   Extending Vessel
Confluent point. Ghost point.

DESCRIPTION

The Kidneys and Bladder are Yin–Yang pairs. The Kidneys are the most Yin organs and they house the most Yin substances. The Bladder is Tai Yang. It distributes the vital substances in the Kidneys throughout the body. Tai Yang is closely related to the Sea of Yang (the Du channel). Both influence Yang and movement. The leg Tai Yang channel can move one on in their life. Shen Mai can assist in moving us forward in life. Along with Zhao Hai, Kidney 6, they are the only confluent points on their channels. Shen Mai helps maintain our stance. This can be our physical stance and movement, or how we stand up for ourselves in dealing with people. Shen Mai can help us extend into the external world, into society, with a good footing and with balance and strength.

TREATMENT

Stimulates and probes the Yang Qiao channel. Removes obstructions from the channel. Enhances movement and agility. Benefits the brain. Shen Mai assists in standing up to others in life interactions. It helps one to explore and interact with the external world. Benefits the eyes. Calms *shen*.

Bladder 61   Pu Can   Subservient Visitor   Servant's Partaking
DESCRIPTION

The Kidneys and Bladder comprise the Water channels and organs, and they correspond to the *zhi*. The Kidneys and Heart are Shao Yin pairs, and the Bladder and Small Intestine are Tai Yang channels. Both the Kidneys and Bladder are connected to the Heart *shen*. A quest in our life is to seek our *shen* and be a living expression of it. The *zhi* and willpower should serve and follow the way of our Heart *shen*. Pu Can can assist in serving the Heart *shen*.

TREATMENT

Influences the way one serves in life. Calms the *shen*, clears the Yang Qiao channel and head.

Bladder 59   *Fu Yang   Instep Yang*

Cleft point.

DESCRIPTION

Yang Qiao reflects our stance in life. This Water channel and the flowing aspect of Water is influenced by Fu Yang. This point assists in moving and getting into the flow of life. Fu Yang can help us stand up and move in life with a balanced stance in life activities and interactions.

TREATMENT

Fu Yang clears obstructions in the Yang Qiao channel.

Gallbladder 29   *Ju Liao   Squatting Bone Hole*

DESCRIPTION

Ju Liao is a major release point for the Yang Wei channel. The Yang Qiao also meets here and it releases both channels. Ju Liao is located at the hip bone. Bones are part of the marrow matrix: Jing, marrow, bones, and the brain. Imbalances can enter this "bone hole" and enter into the marrow level.

TREATMENT

Ju Liao can access and release old patterns and imbalances. Combined with other points on the Yang Wei and other channels, it can release imbalances throughout the body.

Small Intestine 10   Nao Shu   Upper Arm Shu

DESCRIPTION

The upper arm allows movement of the upper limb; Ju Liao, Gallbladder 29, assists in moving the lower limb. Both these points release the Yang Wei and Yang Qiao channels and their energetic properties.

TREATMENT

Nao Shu is a major release point, and assists in bringing out pathogens locally and throughout the body.

Large Intestine 15   Jian Yu   Shoulder Bone

Jian Yu means "shoulder bone."

DESCRIPTION

Jian Yu is the structure to hold and release stresses of life. The Large Intestine is a Yang channel, its intrinsic function is to empty and release. Jian Yu can empty and release stresses and burdens that have accumulated. The Large Intestine channel flows to Da Zhui, Du 14. Jian Yu assists in Da Zhui's ability to raise Yang.

TREATMENT

Jian Yu affects how one can move, both physically and emotionally. Clears stagnations in the Yang Qiao channel.

Large Intestine 16   Ju Gu   Great Bone

DESCRIPTION

Ju Gu influences the scapula, acromion, and clavicle bones (the bones around the shoulder).

TREATMENT

Can release pathogens lodged in the bones around the shoulder. It has a strong influence on structure, posture, and stance, and how we move in life. Clears stagnations in the Yang Qiao channel.

Gallbladder 20   Feng Chi   Wind Pool

The San Jiao pathway crosses here.

DESCRIPTION

Wind can mean change. Understanding change and how to live in harmony with it, is the basis of Chinese philosophy and medicine. The Gallbladder channel is the Wood element, which corresponds to wind and change. When we are rigid, locked, and stagnant, we cannot respond effectively to changes in our environment and changes in our life.

As a point on the Shao Yang channel, Feng Chi can release pathogens that block and stagnate the Shao Yang channel's energetic properties of turning, twisting, bending, adapting, adjusting, and responding.

TREATMENT

Feng Chi releases pathogens that prevent effective interaction with change, which is necessary for healthy decision-making, decisive activity, and the smooth flow of movement in our daily life.

Calms *shen*. Tonifies marrow. Nourishes the brain. Clears pathogenic wind. Helps one adjust to deal with changes in life.

Stomach 4   Di Cang   Earth Granary

DESCRIPTION

Di Cang is the location for postnatal substances to begin the transformation into usable substances for the body. When the *yi* is imbalanced, it influences our relationship to food and eating. Imbalances of the Yang Qiao can include a lack of nourishment and influence our eating habits.

TREATMENT

Di Cang can assist in releasing imbalances in eating patterns from a lack of nourishment manifesting in the Yang Qiao channel. Di Cang assists in digesting postnatal influences.

Stomach 3   Ju Liao   Great Bone Hole

DESCRIPTION

Ju Liao connects the *yi* and *po*, the mouth and the nose. With each breath, life force mixes with the *yi*, the Stomach, and *po* energetic properties. When the *yi* is overactive, when our thoughts are racing and repetitive, it is with soft, gentle, and deep breathing that the *yi* can be brought into the present moment. The breath can calm and root the *yi*. Ju Liao assists in calming the *yi* and repetitive and obsessive thinking.

TREATMENT

Expels wind. Clears obstructions in the channel. Reduces swellings.

Stomach 2   Si Bai   Four Whites

DESCRIPTION

White corresponds to the Metal element, and the Lungs and Large Intestine. Si Bai can influence the Large Intestine and Stomach channels. Located in the foramen, Si Bai is a space that can contain the tears and imbalances of the spirit. It can also guide out the imbalanced energy.

Stomach 1   Cheng Qi   Containing Tears

DESCRIPTION

The eyes are the mirrors of the spirit. The Liver opens to the eyes; the Gallbladder, Bladder, and San Jiao channels all begin near the eye; the Heart flows to the tissues surrounding the eyes. The Large Intestine is the origin of the Stomach channel, and these two Yang Ming channels connect to the eyes. Life influences are contained in our channels and organs, and they flow to the eyes. Cheng Qi can help to release the stresses influencing our life.

TREATMENT

Cheng Qi assists in releasing emotions and stresses; they can come out of the eyes in tears.

Bladder 1 Jing Ming Eye Brightness Eye's Clarity

DESCRIPTION

Jing Ming reflects the eye's ability to see, both physically and in the sense of insight. All channels influence the eyes directly or indirectly, and their qi and condition can be transported to the eyes. "Brightness" can mean the light that reflects the condition of your spirit. It can mean that your inner eye will be involved in fulfilling your destiny, your quest in life. The Bladder is the partner of the Kidneys and the *zhi*. Our will to fulfill our destiny can be perceived in the eyes. In Nei Dan, the inner eye plays an essential role in the cultivation process.

TREATMENT

Influences sleeping. Allows one to see life with clarity. Clears pathogenic factors influencing the eyes. It has a strong relationship to the Qiao channels.

Confluent point (command, opening, master point)

- Shen Mai, Ninth channel, Extending channel, Bladder 62.

Coupled point

- Hou Xi, Back Ravine, Small Intestine 3.

Xi cleft point

- Bladder 59, Fu Yang.

Chapter 13

THE YIN QIAO CHANNEL

Common names
- Yin Heel
- Yin Bridge
- Yin Motility
- Accelerator of Yin
- Yin Walker vessel
- Yin Stance channel

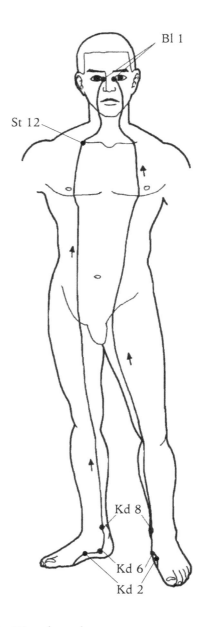

Figure 13.1 The Yin Qiao channel

Internal pathway

The pathway originates from the area of the navicular bone to the medial malleolus at Zhao Hai, Kidney 6. It ascends to the upper portion of the medial malleolus and runs straight upward along the posterior border of the medial aspect of the thigh, to the external genitalia. It then ascends to the abdomen and upward along the chest to the supraclavicular fossa, from where it runs upward lateral to the Adam's apple, through the throat in front of Ren Ying, Stomach 9, and then along the zygoma.

It ascends beside the mouth and nose to the inner canthus, where it meets with the Yang Qiao channel at Jing Ming, Bladder 1, and finally ascends to enter the brain.

Li Shi-Zhen added Ran Gu, Blazing Valley, Kidney 2, to the trajectory.

The Yin Qiao Pathway according to the Pulse Classic

The Yin motility originates within the heel, ascending via the medial malleolus to the throat, where it joins and communicates with the penetrating vessel.

Anatomical areas of influence

The channel influences the inner aspect of the legs, motor impairment of the legs, genitals, abdomen, eyes, brain, *shen*, and the Bladder.

Common conditions the Yin Qiao channel treats

Regulates motion of the lower limb, tightness, and spasm along the medial lower legs with the lateral side of the leg flaccid or atrophied. Controls Yin on the medial and lateral aspects of the body; transports the Yin substances of the lower part of the body to the upper part of the body. Treats pain in the lumbar and hip regions referring to the pubic region, and removes qi and blood stagnation in the genital region. Treats hip and genital pain, pain in the lower abdomen, spasm of the lower limbs, inversion of the foot, hernia, epilepsy, hypersomnia, lethargy, habitual miscarriage, infertility, difficult labor, vaginal discharge, uterine bleeding, diseases of the eyes. Absorbs excess Yin and influences all Yin substances: Yin, blood, fluids, sweat, tears, and nodules.

Yin Qiao channel points and functions

Kidney 2   Ran Gu   Blazing Valley
Spring, Fire point.

DESCRIPTION

Ran Gu is Fire in the Water. It is the Fire or passion that can guide our will to live the type of life we desire.

TREATMENT

Ran Gu can reinforce Kidney Yang. This point is the dragon in the Water, Yang in the Yin, Fire in the Water. It invigorates the Yin Qiao channel. Clears heat, especially false heat.

Kidney 6   Zhao Hai   Shining Sea
Confluent point.

DESCRIPTION

In ancient China, people looked into the sea to see their reflection. The Kidneys are the Water element. Zhao Hai is a portal to see inside our Water, to see our reflection, our true nature. The Kidneys and Water are the most Yin organs, substance, and area of the body. Zhao Hai is a way to see our Yuan Shen. When we are lost, disconnected, lack self-esteem, and no longer trust ourselves, Shining Sea assists in seeing and experiencing our shining spirit. Zhao Hai can influence self-confidence, self-trust, and self-esteem. It allows people to see themselves clearly. Zhao Hai increases the ability to stand up for yourself. Reinforces the Kidneys and the *zhi*.

TREATMENT

Calms the *shen* and the mind. Nourishes Yin, cools blood, and nourishes Water and fluids. Zhao Shen influences the eyes. It regulates the uterus and menstruation.

Kidney 8   Jiao Xin   Intersection Reach
Junction of Faithfulness   Trusting and Good Exchange
Cleft point.

DESCRIPTION

Water can take any shape and form. Its nature is to adapt, join, and interact with everything. Jiao Xin assists in the ability to be open and share. It includes having faith and trust in self and in others. When we have lost faith and trust, Jia Xin can help restore those natural and intrinsic aspects of our life, allowing for smoother interactions and exchanges.

TREATMENT

Jiao Xin stimulates the channel and clears stagnations. This cleft point helps a person move past their current condition. It benefits the uterus and regulates menstruation. The point can be used with Yang Ling Quan, Gallbladder 34, to help a person start moving outward in life.

Stomach 12   Que Pen   Empty Basin

DESCRIPTION

Que Pen is a space that facilitates the flow of substances from Heaven above to Earth below. This space connects the head and chest, and allows for the interaction of the great vessels and innervations in the neck; it also connects the front of the neck to the back of the neck at Da Zhui, Du 14. Stomach 12 can transfer pathogens from all Yang channels, except the Bladder, to Da Zhui. It can also collect pathogens in the neck and the surrounding areas and store them. That can cause certain muscle and skeletal conditions. Many qi gong forms include movements to open this area up, to allow the smooth flow of qi through the head, neck, and chest.

Que Pen connects to Du 14, and facilitates the upright posture. This point and area has a strong downward action; it strongly descends qi. Que Pen allows the heavenly, head qi to flow down. In the Microcosmic Orbit meditation the neck is a major area to let qi flow down the top of the Du channel into the Ren channel.

Bladder 1   Jing Ming   Eye Brightness

Jing Ming reflects the eye's ability to see, both physically and in the sense of insight. All channels influence the eyes directly or indirectly, and their qi and condition can be transported to the eyes. "Brightness" can mean the light that reflects the condition of your spirit. It can mean that your inner eye will be involved in fulfilling your destiny, your quest in life. The Bladder is the partner of the Kidneys and the *zhi*. Our will to fulfill our destiny can be perceived in the eyes. In Nei Dan, the inner eye plays an essential role in the cultivation process.

TREATMENT

Influences sleeping. Allows one to see life with clarity. Clears pathogenic factors influencing the eyes.

Confluent point (command, opening, master point)

- Zhao Hai, Shining Sea, Kidney 6.

Coupled point

- Lie Que, Broken Sequence, Lung 7.

Cleft point

- Jiao Xin, Intersection Reach, Kidney 8.

Chapter 14

THE DAI CHANNEL

Common names
- Belt channel
- Holding channel
- Vessel of Latency
- Sea of Ming Men

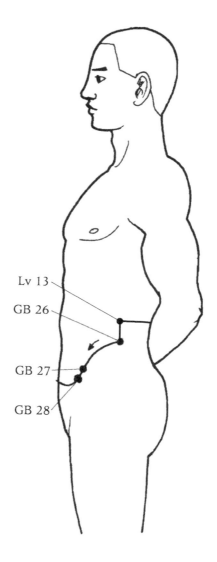

Figure 14.1 The Dai channel

The Dai channel is the belt channel and its location includes the area where a belt is worn. The abdomen is where excesses can be stored. Excesses include physical and emotional conditions, and we can hold on to them for a variety of reasons. For example, we may have suppressed early experiences, or we may feel we don't have the energy or time to deal with them, or we don't want to let them go. When we don't deal with them they can accumulate in the Dai channel and area. A special Taoist abdominal massage, called *Chi Nei Tsang*, focuses solely on the abdomen to release emotions and trauma held. Treating the Dai channel and giving Chi Nei Tsang treatments accomplish the same goal of releasing accumulations and stagnations.

Accumulations in the Dai channel can prevent us from growing, developing, and being creative. The accumulations slow our response to life experiences. We can be limited by the stagnations of the past or by dreams of the future. It takes qi, blood, and Jing, to maintain the excesses. We use our vital substances to maintain these excesses, which drain and weaken us.

Cycles of time relate to the Wei channels, and this is one explanation why the Dai channel is paired with the Yang Wei. The Dai is about not being able to deal with things in the time of now. The Dai channel can release what we have stored, allowing the space to deal with the underlying conditions.

Dampness is a main excess in the Dai channel. The Gallbladder and Liver channels can be involved in the creation of dampness, especially when Wood overacts on Earth. This is the Gallbladder and Liver overacting on the Spleen and Stomach. It is common for stress and emotional disharmony to influence the Gallbladder and Liver to overact, causing damp. If the emotions and stresses are not resolved and released, they can be stored in the Dai channel. When the excesses grow, the Dai can reach the point where it can overflow. The overflow spills out, possibly in the form of discharge. For example, the excesses can be dampness, phlegm, mucus, or blood. The discharge can be emotional as well. Dampness and phlegm can disorient the body by blocking the flow of qi in the channels. The blockages can slow us down in the way we respond to and sync with life.

The Dai and Yang Wei have become a popular channel pairing that can release excesses, especially damp, and with it the inability to respond to life activities. The Wei channels are the linking channels (see Chapter 8), and they and Shao Yang are influenced by damp, a major excess that can block the ability to link, process, make choices, and respond effectively.

Internal pathway

The pathway originates below the hypochondriac region, around the area of Zhang Men, Liver 13. It encircles the area just below the hypochondriac region, running obliquely downwards through Dai Mai, Gallbladder 26, Wu Shu, Gallbladder 27, and Wei Dao, Gallbladder 28, like a belt.

By circling the waist the pathway implies the following points:

1. Liver 13, Zhang Men. Li Shi-Zhen adds this point to the pathway.

2. Ren 8, Shen Que.

3. Kidney 16, Huang Shu.

4. Bladder 52, Zhi Shi.

5. Bladder 23, Shen Shu.

6. Du 4, Ming Men.

The Dai channel pathway according to the Pulse Classic

The Girdle Vessel originates in the region of the free (floating) rib and encircles the body.

Anatomical areas of influence

Gallbladder, Liver, Kidney, Spleen, Stomach, and the Bladder. Divides the body in half: top and bottom, and left and right. Influences the uterus and regulates qi of legs, abdomen, and hips.

Common conditions the Dai channel treats

Distension and fullness of the abdomen, weakness of the lumbar region, gynecological conditions, leucorrhea, prolapse of the uterus, muscular atrophy, weakness and motor impairment of the lower limbs, the hips, dampness, damp in lower Jiao. Regulates qi of Liver, Spleen, and Kidneys.

Dai channel points and functions

Liver 13   Zhang Men   Camphorwood Gate   Order Gate

Spleen *mu.* Influential point of the Fu organs.

DESCRIPTION

Zhang Men has a strong influence on the *yi.* When the *yi* is calm and clear, all the five *shen* and the five Yin organs function efficiently and effectively. Zhang Men brings order and balance to the *yi* and the Spleen and Stomach. When the *yi* is in harmony, Cycle Gate, Liver 14, is in harmony, and a new cycle of health and balance begins. The Dai channel holds pathogens, and when they are not released, Zhang Men can restore order by stimulating the Dai channel to release and let go.

TREATMENT

Zhang Men treats the Liver overacting on the Spleen. It supports the *yi* and the Spleen.

Gallbladder 26   Dai Mai   Girdle Vessel

DESCRIPTION

Dai Mai is on both the Gallbladder and the Dai channels. It is a powerful point to influence the Dai channel and should be considered in Dai channel treatments. The Dai and Shao Yang channels act as filters from the interior and exterior, and above and below. Both channels can release and retain substances, pathogenic factors, emotions, and trauma. The Dai Mai is a powerful point to release what is not needed, and retain what is beneficial.

The belt channel ranges from Dai Mai to Ming Men, Du 4, to *shen* Que, Ren 8, in a circle. The Dai channel influences the Kidneys, Jing, and source qi. Dai Mai can be used to draw Kidney qi to the Gallbladder and Dai channels, to strengthen their energetics. It can also be used to circulate the flow of qi in the lower Dan Tian, to supplement the Kidneys, Jing, and source qi.

TREATMENT

Dai Mai treats gynecological conditions. Resolves damp heat in the lower Jiao. Regulates the uterus.

Gallbladder 27   Wu Shu   Fifth Pivot

DESCRIPTION

The Dai channel in Nei Dan ranges from the bottom of the feet to the top of the head. This channel maintains the integrity of all the channels and structure of the body. Wu Shu assists in maintaining the five major pivots or muscle groups that allow normal structure and movement of the body. The five pivots are the paravertebral, rectus abdominus, occiput, sternocleidomastoid, and gastrocnemius muscles. When our body and mind are flexible, we can be spontaneous and live in tune with the natural rhythms of life. Wu Shu assists in maintaining balance, good posture, and flexibility.

TREATMENT

Treats hernia, uterine prolapse, leucorrhea, and local stagnations.

Gallbladder 28   Wei Dao   Linking Path

DESCRIPTION

Wei Dao clears stagnations and attachments to the past that prevent us from being in the present moment and responding to life in a spontaneous way. Stagnations in the Dai channel prevent us from dealing with cycles of time, which can lead to postponing decisions, and suppressing and repressing feelings, emotions, and stresses. Wei Dao can link or sync us to the rhythms, frequencies, and cycles of the present moment. It can link us to the Dao.

Confluent point (command, opening, master point)

- Zu Lin qi, Foot Overlooking Tears, Gallbladder 41.

Coupled point

- Wai Guan, Outer Gate, San Jiao 5.

Chapter 15

CLINICAL APPLICATIONS OF THE EIGHT EXTRAORDINARY CHANNELS

There is a variety of ways to use the Eight Extraordinary Channels in clinical practice. The following are three common approaches in modern clinical practice.

Constitutional conditions

The Eight Extraordinary Channels are considered the most constitutional channels and have the closest relationship to the Kidneys and Jing. They treat Jing conditions. Jing should be used carefully and for constitutional, chronic, or Yuan level conditions. Using Jing for other conditions would weaken and prematurely deplete essence. To use essence for conditions that Ying and Wei substances can treat would be an inefficient use of the body's vital substances.

Channel conditions

In this method, the Eight Extraordinary Channels are used to treat problems that occur on their pathways. Select points along the pathways to treat the condition.

Polarity conditions

When there are imbalances between sides of the body and their channels, consider using the Eight Extraordinary Channels to balance and harmonize these polarities. These channels and their pairings include left/right and top/bottom point prescriptions.

Qualities of the Eight Extraordinary Channels

The Eight Extraordinary Channels energetic properties are multifaceted and reflect our life. Each channel can be viewed in the following ways:

- Each channel contains prenatal influences and qualities.

- Each channel contains postnatal influences and qualities.

- Postnatal influences can enter the Jing or Yuan level and become part of the constitution.

- Each channel influences physical aspects of the body.

- Each channel influences certain anatomical areas.

- Each channel corresponds to emotional and psychological qualities.

- Each channel has a stronger influence on certain vital substances. For example, the Du channel has a strong influence on Yang and qi, and the Ren channel on Yin and blood.

- Each channel has stronger relationships with certain channels in the acupuncture channel network. For example, the Du channel controls Yang and Wei qi, and has a strong influence on the sinew channels, which is involved with Wei qi.

- The channels can be combined according to numerous principles. There are no definitive channel combinations that are better than others. Combining channels based on their ability to treat the condition is the goal, rather than only using popular combinations.

- Each channel has numerous functions. The objective is to stimulate a channel to perform its function. This objective may require a few points on the channel; one point most likely is not enough. The goal is to sequence points together to stimulate the channel and restore it to its normal function, or restore the channel or organ that is targeted in the treatment. This is the key to creating Eight Extraordinary Channels treatments: combining channels and points to create a synergy.

Diagnostic framework

Learning each of the Eight Extraordinary Channels is the foundation for developing a diagnostic framework for their use in clinical practice. The following four diagnostic methods are guidelines for viewing signs, symptoms, and conditions.

- Diagnosis can be made based on the energetic properties of each of the Eight Extraordinary Channels.

- Diagnosis can be made based on location on the Extraordinary Channel pathways. For example, issues related to the uterus would include the Chong and Ren channels; they originate there.

- Diagnosis can be made based on palpating points and areas along the Eight Extraordinary Channels trajectories. The areas and *ashi* points along the trajectory can be needled. They can be actual Eight Extraordinary Channels points or areas along their pathway.

- Diagnosis can be made based on the relationships between the Eight Extraordinary Channels and vital substances. For example, Ren is the Sea of Yin; body fluids or blood conditions can be treated with the Ren channel. The Du is the Sea of Yang and influences Yang, qi, Wei qi, heat, Fire, and wind.

Applying these guidelines in diagnosis allows for making an Eight Extraordinary Channels treatment plan.

Chapter 16

TREATMENT METHODS

As discussed in the previous chapter, there are a variety of ways to use the Eight Extraordinary Channels in clinical practice. A goal of this book is to provide some approaches to creating treatment plans based on the unique condition of each person. Use these approaches as a guide to customize your treatments.

A comprehensive approach for any treatment

The following treatment approach is a comprehensive method. It can be a guiding approach for any treatment.

1. Select the confluent point of the root problem channel or the predominant channel for treatment. Needle the point on one side.

2. Select a cleft point, if the channel has one.

3. Selecting Eight Extraordinary Channels points on their pathways (trajectories):

   a) Pick points where their function relates to the condition.

   b) Pick *ashi* areas.

   c) Pick a point in the anatomical area related to the condition, for example, near an organ or muscular-skeletal region.

   d) Pick a point near an energy center or vital substances to be treated.

4. Select points from other Eight Extraordinary Channels being used in the treatment.

5. Close the Eight Extraordinary Channels portion of this treatment with the confluent point of the second Eight Extraordinary Channels used in the treatment (if a second one is used in the treatment). Needle the opposite side from the first confluent point. For example, if it was a Chong and Ren channel treatment, begin with Spleen 4 on the left side, and end the treatment with Lung 7 on the right side. If one Eight Extraordinary Channel is used in the treatment, treat the point bi-laterally.

6. Select the confluent point based on gender, and needle one side and then the opposite side of the paired Eight Extraordinary Channels.

   a) For postnatal conditions: The left side is for males and the right side for females. The right is Yin and the left side is Yang.

   b) For prenatal conditions: The left side is for females and the right side for males. Left is Yin and right is Yang.

7. Select relevant points from the primary channels. (Check the case studies in Chapter 18 for examples of this method.) See point 10 in the following section for a pool of common points that could be used with the Eight Extraordinary Channels.

Channel and point selection strategies

1. Select the confluent point only.

2. Combine the confluent point with its Ming dynasty coupled paired point.

3. Combine the confluent point, its corresponding cleft point, and its coupled paired point.

4. Select any combinations of the confluent points based on your diagnostic method, not just the Ming dynasty coupled pairings. Use any combination that fits the diagnosis.

5. Select the confluent point and relevant points along the pathway of the affected Eight Extraordinary Channels. Needle the confluent point, pathway points, and then the closing confluent point.

6. As a strategy, select points that balance upper and lower, and right and left areas of the body. Create a prescription that has a balance of points throughout the body.

7. Select the confluent point, the coupled pair confluent point, and Eight Extraordinary Channels pathway points. Include non-Eight Extraordinary Channels pathway points that are relevant to the condition. For example, if there is essence deficiency, you may select Chong channel points and then add points that reinforce the Kidneys. Some examples of relevant points are Kidney 3, Bladder 23, and Ren 4. These are respectively the source, back *shu*, and a major point to reinforce the Kidneys.

8. Some practitioners needle the confluent-paired points and if the symptoms do not diminish, they select the corresponding sea point. For example, if Spleen 4 is used for the Chong Mai, Spleen 9, the sea point would also be needled.

9. Use the Eight Extraordinary Channels for chronic, deep, or constitutional conditions. Use these channels when there is a condition of the Yuan level, otherwise you are using Jing or source qi to treat conditions that Wei qi or Ying qi could treat.

10. Select points that correspond to the Eight Extraordinary Channels and their energetics, especially Yuan qi. The following are a pool of points to consider in Eight Extraordinary Channels treatments.

    a) source points

    b) sea points

    c) front *mu* points

    d) back *shu* points

    e) San Jiao points (San Jiao is closely related to source qi and Jing)

    f) Kidney points

    g) Gallbladder points

    h) eight influential points

i) divergent channel confluent points

j) four sea points:

- The *Sea of Qi* points affect the amount and flow of qi within the body. These points can be included in conditions related to qi when there is excess, deficiency, or stagnation. The Sea of Qi points are Stomach 9, Bladder 10, Ren 17, Du 14, Du 15.

- The *Sea of Blood* points affect the amount and flow of blood within the body. They can be included in all blood conditions: excess, deficiency, or stagnation. The Sea of Blood points are Bladder 11, Stomach 37, and Stomach 39.

- The *Sea of Grain* points influence the creation of Gu qi and affect digestion. They are Stomach 30 and Stomach 36.

- The *Sea of Marrow* points influence marrow and its related areas of influence. The points are Du 16 and Du 20.

11. When selecting points on the Eight Extraordinary Channels pathways consider:

a) Cleft points on the Eight Extraordinary Channels.

b) Select actual points on the pathway, especially if they are anatomically close to the area of pathology.

c) Select actual points on the pathway that are from the channel involved in the pathology. For example, if the Spleen is part of the pathology, use Spleen 13, Spleen 15, or Spleen 16 from the Yin Wei channel.

d) Use the actual points on the pathways as landmarks, begin there and palpate for *ashi* points and needle them.

e) By needling the confluent point, pathway points, and paired confluent point on the Eight Extraordinary Channels, their pathways and vital substances are stimulated and activated. This begins the process of influencing the Eight Extraordinary Channels.

f) Select points from the primary channels that relate to the treatment.

g) Select points from the sinew and luo channels if the condition is influencing those channels.

12. The Eight Extraordinary Channels are involved with Jing, which includes long cycles of unfolding: the Eight Extraordinary Channels are treating chronic pathologies and patterns, the healing process takes more time than acute conditions, and this level is slow-moving. A person can have a profound experience in one treatment, but it takes time to enter the deeper levels and bring the relevant issue to the attention of the patient. At that time the patient has a choice whether to make the changes necessary for transformation.

13. Combine any combinations of the Eight Extraordinary Channels, not just the Ming dynasty pairings. For example, a treatment for insomnia with chronic dysmenorrhea could include the Yin Wei and Dai channels.

Knowledge of each point on the Eight Extraordinary Channels pathway is a key to optimal usage of these channels in clinical practice.

Combining channel systems

The channel system can be combined in treatment plans. When two or more channels are affected by a condition, or when a channel system is selected to support other channels, multiple channels can be combined in treatments. The following briefly describes how to combine the Eight Extraordinary Channels with other channel systems.

The sinew channels

The sinew channels are used for muscular-skeletal conditions. When there are chronic emotional, postural, or lifestyle conditions that influence the muscular-skeletal system, treat the sinew channels for the pain. Then treat the Eight Extraordinary Channels for the chronic patterns that cause the muscular-skeletal conditions.

The luo channels

The luo channels can treat blood conditions and emotions. Use them to treat emotions, especially for acute emotional conditions. If the emotions are chronic and part of the constitution, consider using the Eight Extraordinary Channels to treat the chronic aspect of the emotions, and use the luo channels for their acute nature.

The primary channels

The primary channels treat the internal organs, and the Eight Extraordinary Channels can be used to support primary channels and the internal organs. The Eight Extraordinary Channels can guide vital substances to the primary channels and the internal organs.

The divergent channels

The divergent channels further the connection of the Yin–Yang paired channels, as well as the Yin–Yang layers of the body (Wei and Yuan layers and qi). These channels can be viewed as a link to all the channels of the body, and can be used to support all channel systems. They can be used with the Eight Extraordinary Channels to treat the organs, by guiding vital substances to them. For example, if there is Kidney Yang deficiency, needle the Du channel to gather Kidney Yang, and the Kidney and Bladder divergent channels to guide the Yang to the Kidneys.

The divergent channels can release conditions latent in the body. For instance, if a person has chronic anger with Liver heat and Fire, treat the Liver and Gallbladder divergent channels to release the chronic energetic pattern, and the Dai channel to help release these energies and patterns.

The divergent channels can also maintain latency. They can be used to guide qi and substances to an area, allowing the body to manage the condition.

Chapter 17

NEEDLING METHODS

The *Nei Jing* presents two main strategies for treatments: reinforcing and reducing. From an acupuncture viewpoint, *to reinforce* means to direct vital substances to an area to supplement, reinforce, tonify, or nourish. Those four words (supplement, reinforce, tonify, nourish) mean the same thing in the practice of acupuncture. Reinforcing means to guide, direct, and move substances to an area. Reinforcing can direct a person to focus on specific areas of their life. If a person suffers from sadness, depression, and grief, a treatment can begin with a release of that condition. After the release, a reinforcing method on channels and points can be applied that direct someone's attention or *yi* to their Heart *shen*, which can attune them with their spirit. *Reducing* means to direct away, release, clear, or sedate. The needling method applied in a treatment determines how the Eight Extraordinary Channels are influenced. By reducing, current intensities can be diminished or released. For example, if a person is very angry from an interaction with a co-worker, applying a reducing method can release them from the emotional intensity of the situation.

Acupuncture points are portals. A portal contains two dimensions: interior and exterior. Every point can be reinforced (guiding inside) or reduced (guiding outside). Needling strategies can be based on several principles; two principles for needling methods are presented here.

The first method is based on the basic function of the organs. Yang organs empty, therefore they are treated to release excess and pathogenic factors. They release both from their own organ and from their Yin–Yang paired organ. Yin organs gather and store. Yin organs are treated to assist in their ability to gather and store. They also store for their Yin–Yang paired organ.

The second method is applying a reinforcing or reducing technique on points, to cause the desired response based on a treatment strategy, not based on the functions of organs.

In the first method, if there was Liver qi stagnation, Gallbladder points would be treated, not Liver points. In the second method, Liver points would be sedated. For instance, a common point to sedate is Tai Chong, Liver 3, for Liver qi stagnation.

There are a few needling techniques for the Eight Extraordinary Channels. Select the methods you feel comfortable with, and consider exploring other methods. A common approach to needling is at the deep level, representative of the Yuan and constitutional level. The needling method should follow the treatment plan.

Needling method

1. Palpate Eight Extraordinary Channels points to activate the point(s), qi, and channel. Then needle the points.

    The *vibrating* and *shaking* technique has been used in the past. The *lifting* and *thrusting* technique is an effective method that mimics the vibrating and shaking technique.

2. Thirty to forty minutes is a common treatment time.

3. Three to six months is a timeframe to evaluate treatments at this level. It takes time to move and transform Jing/essence.

In the *Nei Jing* there are three reinforcing and reducing techniques. These methods are in the *Su Wen*, Chapter 54, "The Art of Acupuncture," and the *Ling Shu*, Chapter 1, "Of Needles and Twelve Source Points," and Chapter 3, "An Explanation of the Minute Needles." Table 17.1 summarizes these methods. Use one or more of the methods in treatments.

TABLE 17.1 REINFORCING AND REDUCING METHODS

Method	Reinforce	Reduce
Respiration	Insert on the exhale	Insert on the inhale
Insertion	Insert slowly, withdraw fast	Insert fast, withdraw slowly
Cover the point	Cover immediately	Cover later

Insertion methods

POSTNATAL PATTERNS BASED ON GENDER

Insert the first needle based on gender. Male is the left side, female is the right side.

PRENATAL PATTERN

Female is the left side and male is the right side.

For genetic or constitutional conditions, consider needling based on prenatal polarity energetic properties.

INFINITY PATTERN

Insert the first needle based on gender. The second point is the paired confluent point. Needle on the opposite side. The third point needled is the same point as the second point; needle it on the opposite side. The fourth point needled is the same point as the first point needled; it is needled on the opposite side. See the example below.

Example for a female

1. Right Small Intestine 3

2. Left Bladder 62

3. Right Bladder 62

4. Left Small Intestine 3

COMPLETION PATTERN

Needle the confluent points bilaterally, and then needle the coupled paired points.

Example

1. Left Small Intestine 3

2. Right Small Intestine 3

3. Left Bladder 62

4. Right Bladder 62

CIRCULATION PATTERN

Finish needling one side of a channel, and then finish the other side. For example, for a Yin Wei channel treatment, needle Kidney 9, Spleen 16, and Liver 14 on the left side, and then treat the same points on the right side.

UNILATERAL CONDITION

Insert the first needle(s) on the opposite side of the condition. For example, if there is a gait issue on the left side of a multiple sclerosis patient, needle the right side first, then needle points on the left side.

Chapter 18

CASE STUDIES

The following case studies are presented as examples of how to select channels and point combinations for Eight Extraordinary Channel treatments. The treatment examples are a guide to assist in creating treatments; they are not meant to be fixed point combinations. The goal is to develop the ability to customize acupuncture treatments to fit your patient's condition. These cases provide guidance on how to think about selecting channels and points. An essential aspect of these treatments is to select a few points on each channel; this will stimulate the entire channel and its energetic properties. The number of points to select will be based on your clinical experience. I suggest two to six points for each channel.

Case 1

A male patient has chronic asthma with difficulty on the inhalation. There is no sputum. There is fatigue, a weak voice, and a pale complexion. The pulse is weak, with a pale tongue.

The diagnosis is Kidney Yang deficiency, the Kidneys unable to hold qi, and Lung qi deficiency. The treatment plan is to reinforce the Kidneys and Lungs by reinforcing the Chong and Ren channels.

1. Spleen 4, left side

2. Stomach 42

3. Stomach 30

4. Kidney 26

5. Ren 4

6. Ren 17

7. Lung 7, right side

Perform an even technique on Spleen 4 and Lung 7. Reinforce all the other points. Angle the needle at Kidney 26 towards the Ren channel.

The patient is a male and the left side is Yang. Insert the first needle on the Yang side. Spleen 4 is the confluent point of the Chong channel. Stomach 42, Chong Yang, is implied on the pathway. It is the source point of the Stomach. Stomach 30, Qi Chong, is the first point on the Chong channel; it is where the pathway flows from the interior of the body to the exterior of the body. This point strongly reinforces essence and the Kidneys. Qi Chong is a Sea of Grain point and also strongly reinforces the Spleen and Stomach. Spleen 4, Stomach 42 and Stomach 30 are on Earth channels, and they reinforce Metal (Lungs). Kidney 26 is the front *shu* point of the Lungs, along with Ren 17; they reinforce the Lungs. Ren 4, Guan Yuan, powerfully reinforces the Kidneys. Lung 7 is the confluent point of the Ren channel.

Consider adding the following points: Kidney 7, Kidney 10, Lung 9. Kidney 7 is the five-phase reinforcing point. Kidney 10 is the sea and horary point, and Lung 9 is the five-phase reinforcing point and the source point of the Lungs.

Case 2

A 72-year-old woman has severe burning urination with dark, scanty urine. She also suffers from a distending sensation at the hypogastrium. The pulse is full, rapid, and wiry, especially in the middle Jiao. The tongue is deep red with a yellow coat. The diagnosis is downward infusion of Liver Fire affecting the Bladder, and damp heat in the lower Jiao. The treatment plan is to clear the Dai channel and Liver Fire.

1. Gallbladder 41, right side

2. Gallbladder 26

3. Bladder 63

4. Gallbladder 35

5. Gallbladder 41, left side

Perform a reducing technique on all points.

Gallbladder 41 is the confluent point of the Dai channel. The right side is selected because it is Yin, and the patient is a female. Gallbladder 26 is Dai Mai, and it is on the Dai channel. Bladder 63 is on the Yang Wei channel and is the cleft of the Bladder. Gallbladder 35 is on the Yang Wei channel and supports releasing the Dai channel. Gallbladder 41 on the left side completes the Eight Extraordinary Channels treatment.

Consider adding the following points: Liver 2, Liver 8, Ren 3. Liver 2 is a spring and Fire point, and clears Liver Fire. Liver 8 is the Water point and clears heat and fluids in the lower Jiao. Ren 3 is the front *mu* point of the Bladder and clears heat by promoting urination.

Case 3

A 54-year-old woman has severe anxiety and claustrophobia. She is anxious when alone at home and has a tight, gripping sensation in the chest. Her pulse is choppy, with a pale tongue and a red tip.

The diagnosis is blood deficiency causing blood stagnation and severe anxiety. The treatment plan is to nourish blood and calm the *shen* with the Yin Wei and Chong channels.

1. Pericardium 6, right side

2. Kidneys 9

3. Spleen 16

4. Liver 14

5. Liver 3

6. Spleen 10

7. Kidney 25

8. Spleen 4, left side

Perform an even technique on Pericardium 6 and Spleen 4. Reinforce Liver 3 and Spleen 10. Reduce Kidney 9, Spleen 16, and Liver 14. Angle the needle on Kidney 25 towards the Ren channel.

Pericardium 6 is the confluent point for the Yin Wei channel, and nourishes Yin and blood and calms the *shen*. It is also Jue Yin and treats the Liver. The right side is Yin and corresponds to females. Kidney 9, Spleen 16 and Liver 14 are on the Yin Wei channel. Combining these three points stimulates Yin Wei energetic properties. Liver 3 and Spleen 10 are implied on the Chong channel pathway and move and nourish blood. Kidney 25 is the front *shu* point of the Heart, combined with Pericardium 6; they create a synergy and calm the *shen*. Spleen 4 is the confluent point of the Chong channel and can be paired with Pericardium 6 and the Yin Wei channel. Spleen 4 is the connecting point and treats blood and emotions.

Case 4

A female has had irregular menstruation for 20 years.

The diagnosis is blood deficiency and blood stagnation. The treatment plan is to activate and nourish blood with the Chong channel.

1. Spleen 4, right side

2. Liver 3

3. Spleen 10

4. Ren 4

5. Ren 12

6. Lung 7, left side

Reinforce all points.

Gong Sun, Spleen 4, is the confluent point of the Chong channel. The right side is Yin and the patient is a female, therefore the right side is needled first. Liver 3, Tai Chong, is on the Chong channel internal pathway. Tai Chong contains the same name as the Chong channel, and is the source point of the Liver. This point reinforces and moves blood. Spleen 10, Xue Hai, the Sea of Blood, reinforces and moves blood. Ren 4,

Guan Yuan, reinforces Yin and blood. Ren 12, Zhong Wan, reinforces the Stomach and the Spleen, and their ability to produce Gu qi and blood. Lung 7 is the confluent point of the Ren channel and closes the treatment. This is a Chong and Ren channel treatment.

Case 5

A 45-year-old man has been in numerous relationships and has been unable to commit to one person. He has always been very independent. He has been in therapy and is thinking about committing to his current girlfriend.

Since this is a chronic bonding condition, the Ren channel is selected. The treatment plan is to nourish Yin and the bonding process.

1. Lung 7, left side

2. Ren 7

3. Ren 12

4. Ren 15

5. Du 20

6. Kidney 6, right side

Reinforce all points.

The left side is Yang and corresponds to males. The first needle is inserted in the left side. Lung 7 is the confluent point of the Ren channel, the Sea of Bonding. Ren 7, 12, and 15 are on the Sea of Yin. These points reinforce Yin and bonding. Yin Jiao, Zhong Wan, and Jiu Wei all direct the treatment internally to the Ren channel. Ren 15 is the source point of Yin; it strongly influences Yin. It is also the luo of the Ren channel, and it can spread this treatment throughout the Yin of the entire body. Du 20 guides the treatment into the Jing-Shen, the brain. Kidney 6 is Shining Sea, it guides the treatment into the Kidneys and the Eight Extraordinary Channels. This nourishes Yin and bonding.

Case 6

A female is turning 50 years old and is overweight. She is having a difficult time dealing with her figure, her shape.

The diagnosis is a Yin Wei condition. The treatment plan is to release the attachment to her body shape, and direct her focus or *yi* on her spirit.

1. Pericardium 6, right side

2. Kidney 9

3. Liver 14

4. Spleen 16

5. Kidney 25

6. Spleen 4, left side

Reduce all points except Kidney 25. Needle Kidney 25 towards the Ren channel. Insert the needle obliquely towards the sternum.

Yin is the right side and Pericardium 6 is the confluent point of the Yin Wei channel, therefore the right side is needled first. Kidney 9 is the cleft point on the Yin Wei channel. It stimulates and moves the channel's energetic properties. Kidney 9 assists in moving the patient from the emotional difficulty about her figure. Liver 14 is Cycle Gate; it is the front *mu* of the Liver. The Liver moves blood and qi, it can move a *yi* that is stagnant. This movement creates a smooth flow of qi and blood, and a free flow of the *yi* to be open to the spontaneity of life. Spleen 16 is Abdominal Lament. This point helps release the *yi* from the patient's repetitive thinking about her figure. Kidney 25 is Spirit Storehouse. It is the front *shu* of the Heart and is used to guide the patient's *yi* on her Heart *shen*. This provides the opportunity for her to refocus her attention on her spirit, not on a false identity. Needling Spleen 4, the confluent point of the Chong channel, finishes the treatment. The Chong channel is the common paired channel with the Yin Wei and is the luo point of the Spleen channel. The Spleen is an Earth organ, and it corresponds to flesh. Luo points treat emotions and Spleen 4 supports treating the *yi*. It can release the emotions related to weight (flesh).

Case 7

A 56-year-old male works in the entertainment industry. He suffers from anger, irritability, and insomnia. This condition has existed for over ten years.

The pulses are rapid and wiry. The tongue body is purple. There is no coating at the tip of the tongue, and it is red. There is a thin, yellow, greasy coat from the middle to the lower Jiao. The diagnosis is Liver Fire, Liver qi stagnation, and damp heat in the middle and lower Jiao.

This is a chronic condition. The treatment plan includes a luo channel treatment to release the emotions. The treatment is Liver 5 on the right side and Gallbladder 37 on the left side. The method is to plum blossom the two points. This pattern matches the polarity of the channels. Liver is a Yin organ and is the right side, and the Gallbladder is a Yang organ and is the left side. These luo points release the intensity of anger and irritability.

After the luo treatment the acupuncture plan is a Yin Wei and Dai channel treatment. The Dai channel is used to release the emotions related to the Liver and Gallbladder. The condition is both acute and chronic; the luo and Dai channel treatment is for the acute emotional condition; the Yin Wei and Dai channels are used to release the patient from old imprints and attachments related to his job.

1. Plum blossom right Liver 5 and left Gallbladder 37

2. Dai channel: Gallbladder 41, 26, and 28

3. Yin Wei channel: Kidney 9, Spleen 16, and Liver 14

Reduce all points.

The luo points release anger, irritability, and heat. Gallbladder 41, 26, and 28 are on the Dai channel, and they release the emotions from a deeper level than the luo channels. Kidney 9, Spleen 16, and Liver 14 are on the Yin Wei channel, and they begin the process of releasing the patient from the chronic patterns generating his current condition.

Case 8

A female patient has chronic back pain in the lumbar area.

The diagnosis is Kidney Yang deficiency. The treatment plan is to tonify the Kidneys with the Du channel.

1. Small Intestine 3, right side

2. Du 4

3. Du 6

4. Du 20

5. Bladder 62, left side

Reinforce all points.

Small Intestine 3 is the opening point of the Du channel. It is also the stream point on the hand Tai Yang channel, and treats the Tai Yang area on the back. Du 4, Ming Men, reinforces Kidney yang. Du 6 is Ji Zhong, Spinal Center. Du 6 guides the treatment into the spine to benefit the marrow matrix and guides the treatment upward towards Du 20. Bai Hui, Du 20, stimulates the brain. This Du channel point combination reinforces the Kidneys and the spine. Bladder 62 is the confluent of the Yang Qiao channel; it supports its Yin–Yang paired channel, the Kidneys. The Bladder channel has an internal pathway that flows into the sacrum and lumbar area. Bladder 62 can move qi and blood, clearing the lumbar area.

Consider adding one or more of the following points: Kidney 3, Kidney 7, Kidney 10, Bladder 16, and Bladder 23. These are the source, five-phase reinforcing and sea points, as well as *du shu* and the Kidney back *shu* point.

Chapter 19

THE POINTS AND NAMES OF THE EIGHT EXTRAORDINARY CHANNELS

1. The Chong channel

Point	Chinese Name	English Name
Ren 1	Hui Yin	Meeting of Yin
Ren 7	Yin Jiao	Yin Junction
Stomach 30	Qi Chong	Penetrating Qi
Kidney 11	Heng Gu	Pubic Bone
Kidney 12	Da He	Great Manifestation
Kidney 13	Qi Xue	Qi Hole, Uterine Gate
Kidney 14	Si Man	Fourfold Fullness
Kidney 15	Zhong Zhu	Central Flow
Kidney 16	Huang Shu	Vital Membranes
Kidney 17	Shang Qu	Shang Bend, Bent Metal
Kidney 18	Shi Guan	Stone Pass
Kidney 19	Yin Du	Yin Metropolis
Kidney 20	Fotong Gu	Abdomen Connecting Valley, Open Valley
Kidney 21	You Men	Dark Gate

The front shu points

The pathway "spreads around the chest." Some view the pathway as ranging from Kidney 22–27 and including the front *shu* points Kidney 22–26.

Point	Intercostal space	Element/organ	Front *shu*	Stomach	Ren
Kidney 22 Bu Lang Corridor Walk	5th	Water Kidneys	Kidney *shu*	18	16
Kidney 23 Shen Feng Spirit Seal	4th	Earth Spleen	Spleen *shu*	17	17
Kidney 24 Ling Xu Spirit Ruins	3rd	Wood Liver	Liver *shu*	16	18
Kidney 25 Shen Cang Spirit Storehouse	2nd	Fire Heart	Heart *shu*	15	19
Kidney 26 Yu Zhong Lively Center	1st	Metal Lungs	Lung *shu*	14	20

2. The Ren channel

Point	Chinese Name	English Name
Ren 1	Hui Yin	Meeting of Yin
Ren 2	Qu Gu	Curved Bone
Ren 3	Zhong Ji	Middle Pole, Central Pole
Ren 4	Guan Yuan	Gate to the Original Qi, Origin Pass

Ren 5	Shi Men	Stone Door, Stone Gate
Ren 6	Qi Hai	Sea of Qi
Ren 8	Shen Que	Spirit Gate
Ren 9	Shui Fen	Water Separation, Water Divide
Ren 10	Xia Wan	Lower Epigastrium, Lower Controller
Ren 11	Jian Li	Interior Strengthening
Ren 12	Zhong Wan	Middle of Epigastrium, Middle Controller
Ren 13	Shang Wan	Upper Epigastrium, Upper Controller
Ren 14	Ju Que	Great Palace, Great Tower Gate
Ren 15	Jiu Wei	Dove Tail
Ren 16	Zhong Ting	Center Courtyard
Ren 17	Tan Zhong	Middle of Chest, Alchemical Altar, Upper Sea of Qi, Chest Center
Ren 18	Yu Tang	Jade Hall
Ren 19	Zi Gong	Purple Palace
Ren 20	Hua Gai	Florid Canopy
Ren 21	Xuan Ji	Jade Pivot, Jade within the Pearl, North Star
Ren 22	Tian Tu	Heavenly Prominence, Opening to the Heavens
Ren 23	Lian Quan	Angular Ridge Spring
Ren 24	Cheng Jiang	Sauce Receptacle

3. The Du channel

Point	Chinese Name	English Name
Du 1	Chiang Qiang	Long Strong, Lasting Strength
Du 2	Yao Shu	Lumbar Shu
Du 3	Yao Yang Guan	Lumbar Yang Gate
Du 4	Ming Men	Gate of Life, Door of Life, Jing Gong, Palace of Essence
Du 5	Xuan Shu	Suspended Axis
Du 6	Ji Zhong	Spinal Center, Adrenal Center
Du 7	Zhong Shu	Central Axis
Du 8	Jin Suo	Tendon Spasm, Sinew Contraction
Du 9	Zhi Yang	Reaching Yang
Du 10	Ling Tai	Spirits Tower, Spirits Pagoda
Du 11	Shen Dao	Spirit Path
Du 12	Shen Zhu	Body Pillar, Spirit Pillar
Du 13	Tao Dao	Middle Path, Way of Happiness, Furnace of the Tao
Du 14	Da Zhui	Big Vertebra, Great Hammer
Du 15	Ya Men	Mute's Gate
Du 16	Feng Fu	Wind Palace, Wind Mansion
Du 17	Nao Hu	Brain's Door
Du 18	Qiang Jian	Unyielding Spine
Du 19	Hou Ding	Behind the Vertex
Du 20	Bai Hui	Hundred Meetings, Hundred Convergences
Du 21	Qiang Ding	Before the Vertex
Du 22	Xin Hui	Fontanel Meeting
Du 23	Shang Xing	Upper Star, Ming Tang, Hall of Brightness

Du 24	Shen Ting	Mind Courtyard, Spirit Court
Du 25	Su Liao	White Bone Hole
Du 26	Ren Zhong	Middle of Person
Du 27	Dui Duan	Extremity of the Mouth
Du 28	Yin Jiao	Gum Intersection

4. The Yang Wei channel

Point	Chinese Name	English Name
Bladder 63, cleft	Jin Men	Metal Gate
Gallbladder 35, cleft	Yang Jiao	Yang Intersection, Yang Convergence
Gallbladder 29	Ju Liao	Squatting Bone Hole
Small Intestine 10	Nao Shu	Upper Arm Shu
Large Intestine 14	Bi Nao	Upper Arm
San Jiao 13	Nao Hui	Upper Arm Convergence
San Jiao 15	Tian Liao	Heavenly Crevice
Gallbladder 21	Jian Jing	Shoulder Well
Gallbladder 13	Ben Shen	Mind Root, Spirit Root
Gallbladder 14	Yang Bai	Yang White
Gallbladder 15	Tou Lin Qi	Falling Tears, Head Overlooking Tears
Gallbladder 16	Mu Chuang	Window of Eye
Gallbladder 17	Zheng Ying	Upright Construction, Correct Plan
Gallbladder 18	Cheng Ling	Spirit Receiver, Spirit Support
Gallbladder 19	Nao Kong	Brain Hollow, Vastness of the Brain
Gallbladder 20	Feng Chi	Wind Pond

Point	Chinese Name	English Name
Du 15	Ya Men	Mute's Gate
Du 16	Feng Fu	Wind Palace, Wind Mansion

5. The Yin Wei channel

Point	Chinese Name	English Name
Kidney 9, cleft	Zhu Bin	Guest House
Spleen 13	Fu She	Bowel Abode
Spleen 15	Da Heng	Great Horizontal
Spleen 16	Fu Ai	Abdominal Lament
Liver 14	Qi Men	Cycle Gate, Gateway of Hope
Ren 22	Tian Tu	Heavenly Prominence, Opening to the Heavens
Ren 23	Lian Quan	Angular Ridge Spring

6. The Yang Qiao channel

Point	Chinese Name	English Name
Bladder 62, confluent	Shen Mai	Ninth channel, Extending Vessel
Bladder 61	Pu Can	Subservient Visitor, Servant's Partaking
Bladder 59, cleft	Fu Yang	Instep Yang
Gallbladder 29	Ju Liao	Squatting Bone Hole
Small Intestine 10	Nao Shu	Upper Arm Shu
Large Intestine 15	Jian Yu	Shoulder Bone
Large Intestine 16	Ju Gu	Great Bone

Gallbladder 20	Feng Chi	Wind Pool
Stomach 4	Di Cang	Earth Granary
Stomach 3	Ju Liao	Great Bone Hole
Stomach 2	Si Bai	Four Whites
Stomach 1	Cheng Qi	Containing Tears
Bladder 1	Jing Ming	Eye Brightness, Eye's Clarity

7. The Yin Qiao channel

Point	Chinese Name	English Name
Kidney 2	Ran Gu	Blazing Valley
Kidney 6	Zhao Hai	Shining Sea
Kidney 8, cleft	Jiao Xin	Intersection Reach, Junction of Faithfulness, Trusting and Good Exchange
Stomach 12	Que Pen	Empty Basin
Bladder 1	Jing Ming	Eye Brightness, Eye's Clarity

8. The Dai channel

Point	Chinese Name	English Name
Liver 13	Zhang Men	Camphorwood Gate, Order Gate
Gallbladder 26	Dai Mai	Girdle Vessel
Gallbladder 27	Wu Shu	Fifth Pivot
Gallbladder 28	Wei Dao	Linking Path
Ren 8	Shen Que	Spirit Gate
Kidney 16	Huang Shu	Vital Membranes

Point	Chinese Name	English Name
Bladder 52	Zhi Shi	Will's Chamber
Bladder 23	Shen Shu	Kidney Shu
Du 4	Ming Men	Gate of Life, Door of Life, Jing Gong, Palace of Essence

Eight Extraordinary Channel pathway points

When considering Eight Extraordinary channel treatments, consider including points from the channels listed in the table below. These channels need to be probed and activated for their corresponding substances and energetic properties to respond to the treatment. The points below are the formal points on the pathways listed in common texts, as well as popular points on the pathway that are not listed in common TCM texts. Consider palpating along the pathway and selecting areas that are sensitive or show abnormal manifestations that reflect pathology.

The Kidney and Gallbladder channels contain the most points.

Channel/ confluent point	Pathway points from major sources
Chong Spleen 4	Spleen 1, Liver 1, Liver 3, Stomach 42, Stomach 36, Spleen 10, Kidney 10, Bladder 40, Stomach 30, Ren 1, Ren 7, Kidney 11–21, Kidney 22–26
Ren Lung 7	Ren 1–24
Du Small Intestine 3	Du 1–28
Dai Mai Gallbladder 41	Liver 13, Gallbladder 26, 27, 28, Ren 8, Ren 4, Kidney 16, Bladder 52, Bladder 23, Du 4
Yin Wei Pericardium 6	Kidney 9, Spleen 13, 15, 16, Liver 14, Ren 22, Ren 23
Yang Wei San Jiao 5	Bladder 63, Gallbladder 35, 29, Small Intestine 10, San Jiao 13, Large Intestine 14, San Jiao 15, Gallbladder 21, Gallbladder 13–20, Du 15, Du 16

Yin Qiao Kidney 6	Kidney 2, 6, 8, Stomach 12, Bladder 1
Yang Qiao Bladder 62	Bladder 62, 61, 59, Gallbladder 29, Small Intestine 10, Large Intestine 15, 16, Gallbladder 20, Stomach 4, 3, 2, 1, Bladder 1, Gallbladder 20

Selecting points by name

Selecting points by name is a powerful way to develop acupuncture treatments. In the table below are some examples of how to organize points by name. Some points have multiple names, which are used in this table. Refer to *Grasping the Wind* (Ellis, Wiseman, and Boss 1989) for names of points. Developing acupuncture treatments based on name, function, and location is a comprehensive method.

Points related to the Chong channel by name

Point	Chinese Name	English Name
Large Intestine 20	Chong Yang	Surging Yang
Stomach 30	Qi Chong	Penetrating Qi
Stomach 42	Chong Yang	Surging Yang
Spleen 12	Chong Men	Surging Gate
Heart 9	Shao Chong	Lesser Surge
Bladder 3	Mei Chong	Eyebrow Ascension Flush/Change
Bladder 4	Bi Chong	Nose Flush
Kidney 1	Di Chong	Earth Thoroughfare
Pericardium 9	Zhong Chong	Central Hub/Thoroughfare
Gallbladder 9	Tian Chong	Celestial Surge/ Hub/Thoroughfare
Liver 3	Tai Chong	Large Surge, Supreme Surge, Great Thoroughfare

Points related to the Du, Yang Wei, and Yang Qiao channels by name

Point	Chinese Name	English Name
Large Intestine 1	Shang Yang	Metal's Note Yang
Large Intestine 5	Yang Xi	Yang Ravine
Small Intestine 5	Yang Gu	Yang Valley
Bladder 39	Wei Yang	Bend Yang
Bladder 35	Hui Yang	Meeting of Yang
Bladder 48	Yang Gang	Yang Intersection
Bladder 55	He Yang	Yang Union
Bladder 59	Fu Yang	Instep Yang
San Jiao 4	Yang Chi	Yang Pool
San Jiao 8	San Yang Jiao	Three Yang Connection
Gallbladder 33	Yi Yang Guan	Knee Yang Joint
Gallbladder 34	Yang Ling Quan	Yang Mount Spring
Gallbladder 35	Yang Jiao	Yang Intersection
Gallbladder 38	Yang Fu	Yang Assistance
Du 9	Zhi Yang	Extremity of Yang

Points related to the Ren, Yin Wei, and Yin Qiao channels by name

Point	Chinese Name	English Name
Stomach 33	Yin Shi	Yin Market
Spleen 6	San Yin Jiao	Three-Leg Intersection
Spleen 9	Yin Ling Quan	Yin Mound Spring
Heart 6	Yin Xi	Yin Cleft
Bladder 14	Jue Yin Shu	Jue Yin Shu
Bladder 67	Zhi Yin	Reaching Yin
Kidney 10	Yin Gu	Yin Valley

Kidney 19	Yin Du	Yin Metropolis
Gallbladder 44	Zu Qiao Yin	Foot Portal Yin
Liver 9	Yin Bao	Yin Bladder
Liver 11	Yin Lian	Yin Corner
Ren 1	Hui Yin	Meeting of Yin
Ren 7	Yin Jiao	Yin Intersection

PART II

THE EIGHT EXTRAORDINARY CHANNELS IN NEI DAN MEDITATION

Chapter 20

THE NEI JING TU

The inner landscape map

The ancient Chinese observed nature by monitoring the activities of the stars, planets, oceans, animal kingdom, seasons, and human behavior. They developed a body of knowledge applicable to lifestyle and medicine. They keenly observed the human body and its inner workings and perceived the relationships between nature and humanity. In their explanations of the relationships they used environmental and cosmic activities as a metaphor for what occurs in the human body. The ancient Chinese drew a diagram called the Nei Jing Tu, the "inner landscape map" (Figure 20.1), to illustrate the inner body structures and functions. The original Nei Jing Tu included landscape designs on the human body, reflecting the inseparable relationship between humanity and nature. (For a guide to the specific points represented in the Nei Jing Tu, see Chapter 26.)

The ancient Chinese healers and Nei Dan practitioners understood life as three-dimensional. They perceived that life could be understood on a physical, psycho-emotional, and spiritual level. The first goal of this section is to share Taoist meditation practices involving the Eight Extraordinary Channels. The second goal is to reveal some of the relationships among the energetics of the Eight Extraordinary Channels, Nei Dan, and Chinese medical energetics. The key to understanding these relationships is the resonances of Heaven, Human, and Earth.

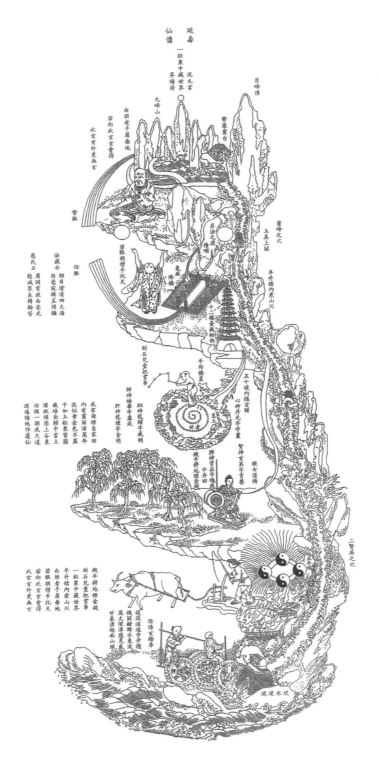

Figure 20.1 The Nei Jing Tu (inner landscape map)

The Resonances of Heaven, Human, and Earth, and the Three Dan Tian

The relationships between nature, humans, and Earth are presented in the *Ling Shu*, Chapter 71. Chapter 71 is called "The mutual resonance between Heaven, Human and Earth." It presents examples of how the ancient Chinese saw resonances of humanity and nature.

- Heaven is round and Earth is flat. A human's head is round and the feet are flat.

- Heaven has the sun and moon. Humans have two eyes.

- Earth has nine regions. Humans have nine orifices.

- Heaven has wind and rain. Humans have joy and anger.

- Heaven has thunder and lighting. Humans have tones and sounds.

- Heaven has four seasons. Humans have four limbs.

- Heaven has the five tones. Humans have five viscera.

- Heaven has winter and summer. Humans have chills and fever.

- Heaven has the ten celestial stems. Humans have ten fingers.

- Heaven has Yin and Yang. Humans have male and female.

- The year has 365 days. Humans have the 365 sections.

- Earth has high mountains. Humans have shoulders and kneecaps.

- Earth has deep valleys. Humans have armpits and creases of the knees.

- Earth has twelve rivers. Humans have twelve major channels.

- Earth has springs and streams. Humans have protective qi.

- Earth has grass and greens. Humans have fine hairs.

- Heaven has day and night. Humans have waking and sleeping.

- Heaven has stars. Humans have teeth.

- Earth has small hills. Humans have small joints.

- Earth has stony mountains. Humans have prominent bones.

- Earth has forest and trees. Humans have muscles.

- Earth has an accumulation of cities. Humans have accumulations of flesh at major joints.

- The year has twelve months. Humans have twelve major joints.

These resonances or correspondences explain insights found in ancient Chinese texts: for example, descriptions of the unity between the human body and the cosmos, as well as the inner functions and unity within the body. These connections are very relevant for a meditation practice called "Nei Dan." Nei Dan means "Inner Pill." A pill or medicine is designed to cause a reaction in the body, to activate body functions. In Nei Dan, we access the deepest aspects of ourselves. The Eight Extraordinary Channels are the links or bridges from your spirit to the external aspects of your life. This linkage is part of us and is always with us. This means you can also access your spirit at any time. A quest in our life is to reconnect or reunite with our spirit, and be a living expression of it. Nei Dan practice assists us in achieving this quest.

The Nei Jing Tu presents the three Dan Tian, and how they are involved with the transformation of Jing to qi to *shen*. It is both a body map and road map. It reveals how the body functions. Moreover, it contains the physical, psycho-emotional, and spiritual qualities that are treated in the practice of acupuncture. The images in the Nei Jing Tu are metaphors. Major relationships to Chinese medicine will be explained, thus providing a roadmap for clinical practice.

There are many qi gong and Nei Dan traditions; most include the three Dan Tian, which are three areas in the body (Figure 20.2). These are sometimes called *Jiao*, "burners" or "centers." "Dan Tian" means energy field. It is an area, not a specific point. Each Dan Tian has organs located in it, which influence different types of vital substances, including types of qi. Through understanding the functions of each we can identify imbalances of organs, vital substances, and emotional conditions. The Nei Jing Tu map shows the three Dan Tian. The Eight Extraordinary Channels are the energy pathways throughout the map. They are the terrain of the map and the body.

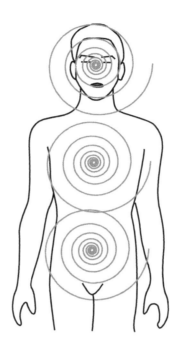

Figure 20.2 The three Dan Tian

The lower Dan Tian ranges from the perineum (the area around the anus) to the coccyx, and up the spine to the Kidneys, where it flows across to the umbilicus, and then back down to the perineum. The lower Dan Tian includes the Kidneys, adrenals, Bladder, sexual organs, pubic bone, pelvis, coccyx, sacrum, and lumbar. The lower Dan Tian influences the processes of the Gate of Vitality. This is the Ming Men cooking Jing, creating source qi (steam). The Kidneys store Jing and the Gate of Vitality. There are two Kidneys: one is Kidney Yang and the other is Kidney Yin. They are the foundation Yin and Yang of the entire body. The Kidneys provide these substances to all other organs. The quality of the Kidneys influences all organs and the entire body.

The middle Dan Tian ranges from the area above the lower Dan Tian to the area of the neck. This Dan Tian includes two energetic influences. The first influence relates to the Spleen and the Stomach. The second influence includes the Lungs and the Heart.

The Spleen and Stomach are the Earth element. The elements and functions of those two organs represent postnatal influences. On a physical level, they include the ability to transform food and drink into energy. On a psycho-emotional level, they correspond to the *yi* spirit. Postnatal influences include the consequences of our actions.

One way to change unfavourable postnatal influences related to the physical body is to change one's diet and exercise. On a psycho-emotional level, the *yi* digests, processes, and organizes our experiences in life. The maturity and refinement of our *yi*, which includes our understanding of life, and the ability to let go of experiences and emotions we do not need, is essential in transforming the imbalances that are created in this Dan Tian. In Chinese medicine, the Spleen holds blood in the vessels, and emotions are stored in the blood. The Spleen holds both blood and emotions. When the *yi* is imbalanced, the Spleen holds emotions that should be let go. This holding creates attachments to emotions, beliefs, and experiences that may create imbalances. Nei Dan cultivation includes resolving imbalances created by the Spleen, Stomach, and the *yi*.

The second aspect of the middle Dan Tian includes the Lungs and the Heart. This area reflects the influences of society. Society includes the conditioning of culture and peer pressure. Those influences can create imbalances that require us to cultivate this area to release from them to obtain balance. This Dan Tian includes the *po* and *shen* of the Lungs and Heart.

The upper Dan Tian ranges from the neck to the crown at the top of the head. The lower Dan Tian represents Earth, the middle Dan Tian represents Humanity, and the upper Dan Tian represents Heaven. The upper Dan Tian represents our connection to our Yuan Shen/original spirit (Heaven). By transforming the lower and middle Dan Tian, we are ready to connect to our spirit. When we connect to our spirit, we are connected to the Tao. Imbalances in the lower and middle Dan Tian can create the illusion that this connection does not exist. Nei Dan is one way to assist people in their self-realization of their spiritual nature.

The Eight Extraordinary Channels play an essential role in understanding the types of stagnations and blockages that manifest in the three Dan Tian, and in our life. This book presents qualities about each of the channels and provides the foundation for treatments and practices to balance them, including acupuncture and Nei Dan.

Jing is our prenatal essence and creates Yuan qi/source qi. It also contains our genes and ancestral influences. The ability of the lower Dan Tian to function properly is essential for the Kidneys' ability to generate source qi. Nutrition, exercise, and a healthy lifestyle have a favorable effect on the Kidneys and their functioning. Stress, lack of exercise, poor diet, and excess sexual activity can drain Jing, and weaken the Kidneys. A major aspect in obtaining health, vitality, and longevity is to live a lifestyle that supports the Kidneys, which will support our foundation. Nei Dan directly influences the functions of the lower Dan Tian and the Kidneys.

Taoist philosophy is Earth-based. It contains a deep connection to Earth and Water. This connection includes the energetics, as well as the functions and movements, of both Earth and Water. Water is the element of highest abundance on our planet, and likewise in our body. The Chinese include Water in their explanation of Chinese medicine. The observation of the flow of seas, rivers, streams, springs, and wells, revealed how their country was nourished with Water. Smooth flows of Water brought bountiful harvests to agriculture, and life to humanity. Excesses, stagnations, blockages, and deficiencies in Water flow caused flooding, drought, decay, and illness. The distribution of Water throughout the country was seen as a model to be applied to the human body. Ancient healers viewed the flow of vital substances in the body as a mirror of the flow of Water throughout a country. Since efficient Water flow is essential for bountiful harvest, and since the drinking of Water is essential for life, the flow of vital substances throughout the body is essential to health. Stagnations, deficiencies, or abnormal flows of vital substances cause illness. This circulatory model is fundamental to the function of the body. In Nei Dan, we implement this imagery of Water circulation.

Chinese medicine includes descriptions of circulation patterns of vital substances. The acupuncture channel system is a pathway for their circulation. The terrain covered by the channels is the landscape. The channels include the sinews, luo, primary, divergent, and Eight Extraordinary Channels. There are qi gong forms that influence each of these channels. The Eight Extraordinary Channels pathways are presented in this book. They are where we perform our Nei Dan practice. The pathways are part of the inner landscape.

The Eight Extraordinary Channels are links to the deepest aspects of the three treasures: the physical, psycho-emotional, and spiritual. They can access the spiritual aspects of our life. They are the bridge from the deep to the superficial. When these channels are clear and free flowing, we are in a high frequency. Each of the three treasures has its own vibration or frequency. The conditions presented in Part I of this book indicate if there are imbalances in the channels, areas, or organs in the body. By practicing Nei Dan, we can cultivate these areas without the need for acupuncture or herbs. However, by combining two or three of these (i.e. Nei Dan, acupuncture, herbs), we can create a powerful synergy.

In qi gong and Nei Dan, there is an important principle: where the mind or intention goes, qi will follow. Wherever we move our intention or focus, qi will follow. Mind guides qi. In our Nei Dan practice of the Eight Extraordinary Channels, we move our intention through the channels, as a means to clear, vitalize, and rejuvenate them. As these channels and qi are refined, we are able to move from "heavy energy" to "light energy." We are converting Jing to *shen*. The Nei Jing Tu diagram shows this refining process. There are circles throughout the Microcosmic Orbit. They flow in a loop from Hui Yin (at the perineum), up the Du channel to the crown, and then back down the Ren channel to the perineum. These circles are yellow, black, or a mixture of the two. Black/dark is Yin and yellow/clear is Yang. At the most Yin area of the body, the perineum, the circles are all dark. Moving up the spine and Du channel, gradually the circles become more yellow. When they reach the crown, the circle is all yellow. The circles indicate the Yin and Yang areas of the body, and the transformation of Yin to Yang, or Jing to *shen* (see Figure 21.1).

Life is comprised of variations of qi. Qi can be dense or subtle. Qi in dense form is Jing. Qi in subtle form is *shen*. Each variation of qi contains a vibration or frequency. Each of the three Dan Tian contains organs that produce a unique qi in its area. The three Dan Tian are slightly different from a Chinese medical viewpoint compared to the Nei Dan viewpoint.

- The lower Dan Tian includes the Kidneys, and they produce Yuan qi (source qi).

- The middle Dan Tian contains the Spleen and Stomach, and they produce Gu qi (nutritive qi).

- The upper Dan Tian contains the Lungs and Heart, and they produce Zhong qi (gathering qi).

The three types of qi support the unfolding of Jing to *shen*. The qi part of Jing–qi–*shen* comprises each of the three treasures, and is the force guiding their unfolding from dense to subtle, from Jing to *shen*. The Nei Jing Tu contains images reflecting the type of transformations that occur in each

Dan Tian. The role of the three Dan Tian in human transformation, and *shen* realization, is explained within the Nei Jing Tu.

A definition of alchemy would include: *Alchemy is making a conscious effort to change.* The Nei Jing Tu and Nei Dan are the map and directions for change. The type of change that occurs is a shift from one's current state to alignment with *shen*. A quest in our life is to seek and realize our original nature, our spirit, and to live from it. Unifying the insight of the Nei Jing Tu with the acupuncture system provides a profound means to assist people in this quest.

Nei Dan begins by relaxing. Only by relaxing can the body begin to let go of stress and allow the normal circulation of vital substances throughout the body. This normal circulation begins the process of clearing imbalances, and energizing and rejuvenating the body, mind, and spirit.

Relaxing with the inner smile meditation

A wonderful way to begin a Nei Dan practice is with the inner smile meditation. This meditation generates a relaxing energy and it can be practiced before the Microcosmic Orbit (Heavenly Orbit).

Inner smile meditation part 1

- Begin by sitting on a chair or on the floor. Your spine should be straight. Place the tip of your tongue at your palate (the roof of the mouth).

- Hold your hands in your lap in any way that is comfortable for you.

- Begin by smiling for a few minutes. When you feel relaxed, continue to smile, and place your mind's attention at the top of your head. Continue to smile throughout the entire meditation.

- Smile as you move your attention down the front and back of your head, and continue down to your neck.

- Continue smiling down your neck to your chest, and then down to the groin and down the back to the lumbar area. Continue moving down your legs to your toes. Continue to smile throughout the meditation.

- Gently move your attention to your shoulders and smile down your arms. Take as much time as you need until you feel relaxed and a smiling energy.

- Gently bring your attention to the Heart center (between your nipples, behind the sternum). Smile into the Heart center and repeat the words "smiling, loving energy." Continue at the Heart center until you feel energy. This part of the meditation may last a few minutes. When you feel a smiling/loving feeling, you can move to part 2.

Inner smile meditation part 2

- When you feel the smiling, loving energy at the Heart center, move your attention to your Heart. Repeat the words "joy" and "love." Feel joy and love in your Heart. Do this for one to five minutes, or until you feel joy and love.

- When you feel joy and love in your Heart, move your attention into your Lungs. Smile and repeat the word "courage." Feel courage in your Lungs. Do this until you feel the energy.

- When you feel energy in your Lungs, move your attention to your Liver. Smile and repeat the word "kindness." Feel kindness in your Liver. Do this until you feel energy in your Liver.

- When you feel energy in your Liver, move your attention into your Spleen. Smile and repeat the word "openness." Feel openness in your Spleen. Do this until you feel the energy in your Spleen.

- When you feel energy in your Spleen, move your attention to your Kidneys. Smile and repeat the word "gentleness." Feel gentleness in your Kidneys. Do this until you feel energy in your Kidneys.

Finish this meditation by gently moving your attention to the center of the lower Dan Tian (behind and below the navel). Focus there for three to five minutes. After completing the meditation, open your eyes and stretch and enjoy. If you are going to continue with more Nei Dan practice, gently move on to the Microcosmic Orbit.

Chapter 21

INNER MEDITATION ON THE REN AND DU CHANNELS
THE HEAVENLY ORBIT

The Nei Jing Tu is a map of the body. It includes major channels, organs, and energy centers of the body. The Ren and Du channels comprise a circuit that flows up the back of the body and then down the front of the body. This circuit has a few names, for example, the "Heavenly Orbit," the "small Heavenly Orbit," the "Orbit" and the "Microcosmic Orbit." The Chinese name is Xiao Zhou Tien.

Figure 21.1 is a modern version of the Nei Jing Tu. This diagram includes the Heavenly Orbit and the three Dan Tian. It is a good image to guide the Microcosmic Orbit Nei Dan practice. The chapters in Part I on the Ren and Du channels present their pathways, functions, and energetics. Nei Dan inner meditation practice clears the channels and assists in opening blockages in the channels. It energizes the channels by circulating your *yi*, or attention, in them. Since planets are constantly circulating in their patterns in space, this orbit reflects the importance of circulation. Lifestyle, poor diet and posture, and emotional imbalances can cause blockages in this orbit. By practicing Nei Dan we can clear, cleanse, and energize these core channels. The efficiency of the functioning of the Sea of Yin and the Sea of Yang channels creates a direct influence on all the Yin and Yang substances and channels in the body.

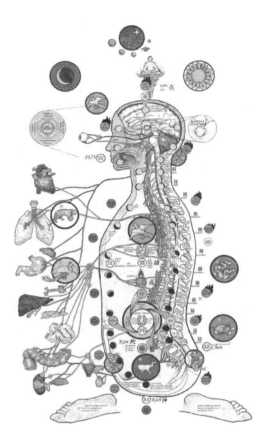

Figure 21.1 The modern Nei Jing Tu

The center

Life begins in the lower Dan Tian. Therefore, we begin Nei Dan in the lower Dan Tian. This Dan Tian is the center of the body. It is the root and the foundation. The lower Dan Tian is often called the "Sea of Qi." It is the origin of source qi. It is the origin of Kidney Yin and Kidney Yang. These vital substances ignite, fuel, and vitalize the entire body. We begin our practice by focusing our attention in the Sea of Qi. Wherever we focus our attention, qi moves to that area. The Spleen has the ability to focus and concentrate. In qi gong theory, "focusing our attention" is under the control of the Spleen and the *yi*. Focus guides qi. When focusing in the lower Dan Tian, qi will be directed there. As qi fills the lower Dan Tian, it energizes the area. It energizes the organs, the glands, and all of the functions of the area. This begins the process of regenerating the area. The entire body benefits when the lower Dan Tian is regenerated and rejuvenated.

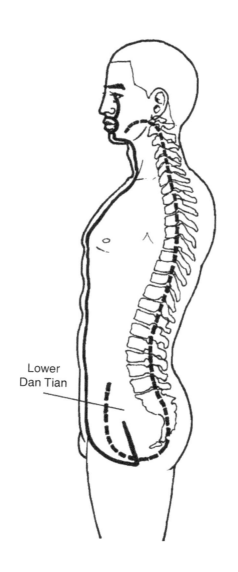

Figure 21.2 The lower Dan Tian

The location to focus our attention in the lower Dan Tian can vary. It is commonly described as behind the umbilicus and one to three inches below it. This is the approximate area. My suggestion is to place your attention in this area and move your attention around until you feel something. It can be a feeling of fullness, tingling, denseness, energy, or a pull. The location can change from day to day. Feeling guides the location. Feeling will be the guiding principle behind the entire practice. If you do not feel anything, continue with one of the methods, and with time and practice you will feel the qi.

The body has a built-in circuit system which includes the Eight Extraordinary Channels. As the lower Dan Tian fills with qi, it is restored to a level of homeostasis or balance. As this area fills up, qi will move throughout the body according to a built-in intelligence. Nei Dan is a way to enhance the flow of qi through the body. It will clear blockages, reduce excesses, supplement deficiencies, and rejuvenate the body. It can accelerate the process of rejuvenation.

Beginning Nei Dan

Nei Dan begins with being centered and relaxed. A way to allow this feeling to occur is by focusing attention in the lower Dan Tian. There are a few ways to practice this focusing, a couple of which are now described.

Method 1: Focusing

Begin by focusing on a fixed point or area within the lower Dan Tian. Keep your attention on the area as you breathe naturally. Inhaling draws qi to the area. Exhaling retains the qi. This process of keeping attention on an area gathers and retains qi to the area, filling it up with qi. As the Sea of Qi is filled with qi, it naturally flows through the body. Practice this cultivation for one, two, three, five, eight, ten, or even twenty minutes. There is no hurry. Build up the length of your practice in a comfortable way.

Method 2: Spiraling

A second method is based on spiraling. The Taoists were cosmologists. They observed the stars and planets, and they noticed that they flowed in predictable patterns. Often we do not notice the most obvious activities around us. Earth is a planet floating in space, and since it is constantly spinning and moving in space, it is always in movement. Guided by the flow of the stars and planets, the ancients turned their attention inward and could feel qi moving in their body. They practiced methods to enhance internal spinning and circulation.

Spiraling causes qi to move to an area. Spiraling gathers, collects, and accumulates qi. Spiraling is a way to move qi; focus is a way to guide qi. Combining both of these is a way to gather and guide qi. Spiraling can be combined with Method 1 of Nei Dan meditation. Begin by focusing attention in the lower Dan Tian. Then after a minute or two, begin spiraling by visualizing a point that is spiraling within a space the size of a marble or a pearl. You can spiral clockwise or counter-clockwise. You can mix the directions up; move in one direction, then the other direction. You can spiral until you feel the qi. Spiraling is commonly done in multiples of three. It can be 9, 18, 27, or 36 times. Do this in both directions, and do it until you feel qi. Be consistent in your spiraling. If you spiral 9 times in one direction, then spiral 9 times in the other direction.

Perform this practice until you feel qi. Select one method or combine the two: you can do only the focus method, only the spiraling method, or a combination both methods. Practice this part of Nei Dan until you feel qi in the lower Dan Tian, which can take from a week to a few months.

The Microcosmic Orbit

Refer to the diagrams in the chapters on Nei Dan, as well as the channel pathways throughout the book, to get a clear understanding of the areas they flow through, which will be where you practice Nei Dan.

The Microcosmic Orbit is the circuit consisting of the Du and Ren channels (Figure 21.3). This Nei Dan practice has you guide your focus from the center of the lower Dan Tian, down to the Hui Yin point, which is the perineum, or about an inch above the anus. From Hui Yin, guide your attention or *yi* up to the crown, to the Bai Hui point. This process guides attention up the Du channel. The next step is to guide your focus down the front of the body and back to the Hui Yin point at the perineum. In so doing, your attention has been guided down the Ren channel. Having returned to Hui Yin, you have completed one circuit through the Microcosmic Orbit (see Figure 21.3).

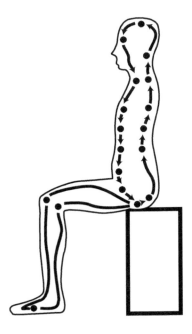

Figure 21.3 The Microcosmic Orbit

There are various ways to practice this Nei Dan. Three methods are presented below. The first way is to connect the circulation up the Du channel and down the Ren channel with your breath.

The first Microcosmic Orbit method

1. Throughout this Nei Dan, your breathing should be natural, relaxed, and gentle. Breathe from your lower Dan Tian.

2. Begin by connecting to the center/the lower Dan Tian. Focus and/ or spiral in the center until you feel qi.

3. Inhale gently into the center. Stay relaxed, and do not change the rate of your breathing. Exhale, and gently move your attention to the Hui Yin area at the perineum.

4. From the Hui Yin area, inhale up the Du channel (in front of the spine) as you count "one." Gently guide your mind up the Du channel to the crown (Bai Hui point). Review the picture of the orbit to visualize the area up the back channel.

5. The inhale should be completed when you arrive at the crown, at the top of the head.

6. Next, guide your focus/attention down the Ren channel. Thus, during the exhale guide your attention from the crown to Hui Yin. Think the number "two," as you flow down the front channel.

7. Yang numbers are odd and they ascend. Count an odd number as you inhale up the back (the Du channel). Yin numbers are even and they descend. Count an even number as you exhale down the front of the body (the Ren channel).

8. Continue this circulation up the back and down the front for ten cycles. This completes one round.

9. Repeat this practice for three, six, or nine rounds. Do it until you feel the qi flowing in the heavenly orbit.

A goal of the Nei Dan is to increase the flow of qi in the channels. Attention or focus guides qi. Moving your attention up the Du and down the Ren increases qi flow in the channels, and assists in breaking through any stagnations or blockages. This process increases energy and refines your qi. Consistent practice strengthens the internal organs, the glands, and the brain. It also refines your Jing to qi and *shen*. Consistent practice draws Jing from the Yin area of the body up to the crown. The lower Dan Tian reflects Yin and Jing, and the upper Dan Tian represents Yang and *shen*.

Gathering qi

Gathering qi at the end of each Nei Dan practice is essential to build, store and rejuvenate the body. There are various methods of gathering and storing, two of which are described below. Select the method that you feel is more effective. You can alternate or mix the methods.

SPIRALING TO GATHER QI

When finishing the practice, gently bring your attention to the center of the lower Dan Tian. In the center, repeat the method used at the beginning of the practice. With your attention, spiral in clockwise and counter-clockwise directions; spiral in cycles of 9 or 18 in each direction, until you feel qi gathering. The range of your spiraling can be the size of a silver dollar or a pearl. If you feel the need to expand the size, you can do it. When you finish spiraling, gently stop and keep your attention fixed in the center in the lower Dan Tian.

An alternative method to finish the practice is to bring your attention to the center of the lower Dan Tian, and then keep it fixed as you inhale and exhale. With your mind fixed in the center, each inhale draws qi there and each exhale stores qi. As you fill the center with qi, you fill the origin point of the Eight Extraordinary Channels. This qi will flow into all the channels, rejuvenating the body.

The second Microcosmic Orbit method

In this method, guide your attention/*yi* up the Du and down the Ren without connecting the circulation to your breath or counting. Circulate through the orbit at a comfortable pace. Continue the circulation through the orbit until you feel qi. Complete this meditation by gathering and collecting qi in the center of the lower Dan Tian.

The third Microcosmic Orbit method

In this method, bring your attention to major points or centers along the Heavenly Orbit (listed below). Begin by focusing your attention below and behind the navel. Spiral clockwise and counter-clockwise until you feel qi. The spiraling can be based on numbers (for example, multiples of nine is good) or until you feel qi. Stay balanced in the amount of clockwise and counter-clockwise spiraling. When you feel qi, gently move to the next point on the orbit and repeat the process.

Continue this process for all the major points on the orbit. It may take time to open all the points. Begin by circulating through the orbit, work on some points, and then continue circulating through the orbit. Close the meditation in the normal way by gathering and storing qi in the center in the lower Dan Tian.

Always begin in the order listed below. You can try one or two points, then circulate through the orbit, and finally close by gathering qi in the lower Dan Tian. There is no rigid rule as to how many points to work on in one sitting. Be flexible.

POINTS ALONG THE HEAVENLY ORBIT

Begin by finding the center (near the navel) in the lower Dan Tian. The center can range along the points and areas listed below. The range is from the navel to a few inches below and inside the body.

- *Navel*
  - Shen Que, Ren 8
  - Qi Hai, Ren 6
  - Guan Yuan, Ren 4
  - Zhong Ji, Ren 3
- *Perineum*
  - Hui Yin, Ren 1
- *Coccyx*
  - Chang Qiang, Du 1

- *Lumbar 2*
  - Ming Men, Du 4
- *Thoracic vertebra 11*
  - Ji Zhong, Spinal Center, Adrenal Center, Du 6
- *Thoracic vertebra 5*
  - Shen Dao, Spirit Path, Du 11, opposite the Heart
- *Cervical vertebra 7*
  - Da Zhui, Big Vertebra, Du 14, opposite the throat
- *Cervical vertebra 1*
  - Ya Men, Gate of Muteness (Jade Pillow), Du 15
- *Crown*
  - Bai Hui, Hundred Meetings, Du 20
- *Third eye*
  - Yin Tang, Mid-Eyebrow
- *Palate*
  - Hsuan Ying, Heavenly Pool
- *Throat*
  - Tian Tu, Heaven's Chimney, Ren 22
- *Heart center*
  - The location is at the fourth intercostal space behind the sternum
  - Tan Zhong, Ren 17

- *Solar plexus*

  ◦ Zhong Wan, Middle of the Stomach, Ren 12

- *Umbilicus*

  ◦ Shen Que, Ren 8

After opening point(s), circulate qi through the orbit, and then close by gathering qi in the center of the lower Dan Tian. Smile throughout the meditation.

※

Some Nei Dan traditions have females (or alternate males and females) circulating up the Ren channel and down the Du channel. This is circulating up the front channel and down the back channel in the Microcosmic Orbit. I use both methods. I may start up the back and down the front, and then practice up the front and down the back channel. I finish by circulating up the back channel and down the front channel. Continue circulating in directional flow until you feel qi. Circulating in both ways can assist in balancing the Yin and Yang energies in the body. Follow how you feel. Always be guided by your feeling. Complete the meditation by gathering qi in the center of the lower Dan Tian.

Chapter 22

INNER MEDITATION ON THE WEI AND QIAO CHANNELS

The Eight Extraordinary Channels Nei Dan includes guiding qi through those channels and areas of the body. The Eight Extraordinary Channels are big channels; they are like seas, not streams. They cover large aspects of the body. The Wei channels were added to the body of Chinese medicine after the early Han dynasty classics, and they are close to the Qiao channels. Viewed as large seas, the Qiao and Wei channels can be combined in this Nei Dan.

Yang Wei and Yang Qiao practice 1: From feet to hips

This cultivation begins with the lateral aspects of the legs: the Yang Wei and Yang Qiao channels (see Figure 22.1).

This meditation starts in the center of the lower Dan Tian, the origin of life and the Extraordinary Channels. From the center our attention is guided through the Heavenly Orbit: the Du and Ren channels. After these core channels are open and you feel the qi flowing, move your focus to the leg channels: the Yang Wei and Yang Qiao channels. Notice the locations of the beginning of the two channels; they originate at the lateral aspect of the foot.

Move your attention from the center over to the hips, and then down the lateral aspect of the legs, to below the lateral ankle. Place your attention at the external part of the foot. As you inhale, move your mind up to the hips. Then exhale back down the lateral part of the legs to the feet. Trace the areas shown in Figure 22.1. Repeat this process 9 or 18 times (until you feel the qi). This clears and energizes the channels.

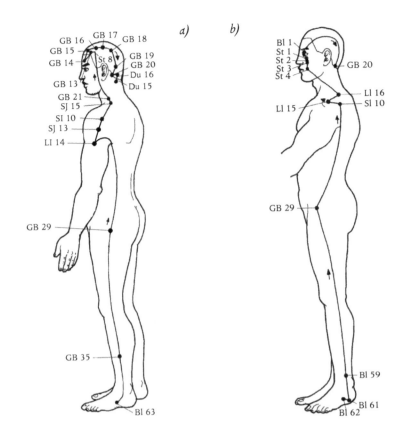

Figure 22.1 a) The Yang Wei channel and b) The Yang Qiao channel

This meditation can be practiced on one side followed by the other, or it can be practiced on both sides at the same time. You can go on to the Yin Wei and Yin Qiao channels, or end the meditation by gathering qi in the center of the lower Dan Tian.

Yin Wei and Yin Qiao practice 1: From feet to hips

Once qi is felt in the Yang Wei and Yang Qiao channels, move to the Yin Wei and Yin Qiao channels (see Figure 22.2). Repeat the process already practiced on the Yang Wei and Yang Qiao channels. Begin by bringing your attention to below the medial ankle at the bottom of the feet. As you inhale, guide your attention up the inner thighs to the pubic bone. Time your inhale so that it finishes as you reach the pubic bone. Exhale as you guide your attention back to the inner legs, to the starting point. Repeat this practice of inhaling up the legs and exhaling down the legs, for a cycle of 10 times. Continue practicing in sets of 10 until you feel qi.

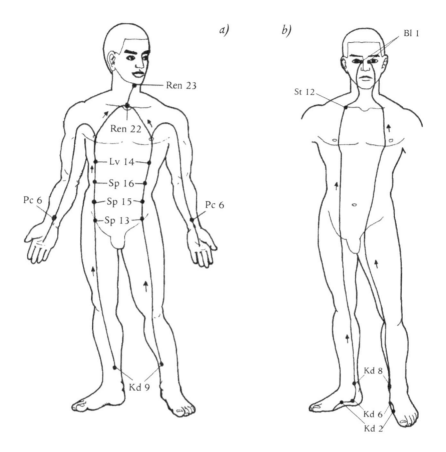

Figure 22.2 a) The Yin Wei channel and b) The Yin Qiao channel

Yang Wei and Yang Qiao practice 2: From hips to brain

This practice continues from the previous Yang Wei/Yang Qiao practice, expanding beyond the hips and flowing up the channels along the sides of the body to the shoulders, neck, head, and brain. The practice begins at the bottom of the foot. As you inhale, guide your attention up the body to the hips, sides of the body, shoulders, neck, front of the face, around the temples, and to the occipital area and into the brain. This should be a soft, gentle inhale, connected with the process of guiding your attention and qi along the channels into the brain. As you exhale, guide your attention back down the channels to the bottom of the feet. One round is five inhales and five exhales. Repeat rounds until you feel qi in these channels.

Yin Wei and Yin Qiao practice 2: From hips to brain

Continuing from the previous Yin Wei/Yin Qiao practice, begin below the inside of the ankle at the bottom of the feet, and inhale up past the pubic bone to the abdomen, the chest, neck, face, eyes, and finally into the brain. This flow is the pathway of the Yin Wei and Yin Qiao channels. More specifically, begin with your attention below the inside of the ankles at the bottom of your feet and gently inhale from the bottom of the feet up the inner leg, abdomen, chest, neck, along the face, to the eyes and into the brain. Gently exhale back down to the bottom of the feet. Repeat the cycle of up and down these channels: 10 times is one round. Repeat rounds until you feel qi in these channels.

Cultivating the Wei and Qiao channels is a way to clear the channels of stagnations and blockages. This practice creates waves of qi that energize the channels. The stagnations, blockages, and old patterns may be conditions presented in Part I of this book.

Chapter 23

INNER MEDITATION ON THE DAI CHANNEL

The Dai channel is the "belt channel." It is a unique channel because it is the only horizontal channel of the Eight Extraordinary Channels. It connects the right and left sides of the body, as well as the upper and lower areas of the body; it unifies all the channels and areas of the body. From a Nei Dan perspective, it has four major functions: it connects the left and right sides, the upper and lower, and the interior and exterior areas of the body, and it is also a protective shield from the exterior. It is a Wei qi field.

The Dai channel plays an important role in filtering. This filtering process includes all the Eight Extraordinary Channels, as well as the interior and exterior of the body. A belt holds things in; this channel can hold things. The things it can hold include emotions, trauma, and pathogenic factors. When the belt channel is not functioning properly, pathogens are held which can create more imbalances and stresses on the body. It is essential to clear the belt channel to allow proper filtering in the body. The belt channel is also a protective qi field that protects from exterior factors, for example wind, cold, and heat. It also protects against influences from other people. Clearing the belt channel helps the effective filtering of pathogens and life experiences. It helps to keep what is beneficial, and to let go of what is not healthy.

In acupuncture theory, the Dai channel has a narrow pathway. In qi gong and Nei Dan, it is a pathway that covers the entire body (see Figure 23.1).

Dai channel Nei Dan part 1

The Dai channel Nei Dan begins in the lower Dan Tian. This meditation connects the front, right, back, and left aspects of the body. It also connects the Ren and Du channels.

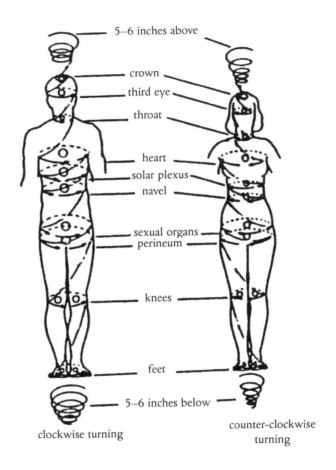

Figure 23.1 The Dai channel

After practicing the Microcosmic Orbit and the Wei/Qiao channel meditations, begin by bringing your attention to the center of the lower Dan Tian. After you feel qi, move your attention in a clockwise circle inside the body at the level of the umbilicus/Shen Que, Ren 8. Spiral an inch or two inside the body. Spiral until you feel qi. Spiral 9 times clockwise and then 9 times counter-clockwise, until you feel qi. You can spiral 18 times or more in each direction. With practice, the qi feeling will arrive faster. This spiraling or spinning process continues at 9 different levels in the body, as well as below the feet and above the head. Spiral counter-clockwise as you ascend, and clockwise as you descend these levels. The order of the levels is as follows:

1. Navel Center, Shen Que, Ren 8

2. Solar Plexus Center, Zhong Wan, Ren 12

3. Heart Center, Tan Zhong, Ren 17

4. Throat Center, Ren Ying, Stomach 9

5. Third Eye Center, Yin Tang

6. Crown Center, Bai Hui, Du 20

Move your focus to a point a few inches above your head, and spiral for a few seconds, then descend clockwise in long spirals, from Du 20 to the perineum.

7. Perineum, Hui Yin, Ren 1

8. Knee Center, Wei Zhong, Bladder 40

9. Ankle Center, Tai Xi, Kidney 3 and Shen Mai, Bladder 62

Move your focus to a point a few inches below your feet, and spiral for a few seconds. Then spiral from below the feet in a counter-clockwise pattern from below the feet to above the head. Repeat this descending and ascending spiralling 3, 6, or 9 times, until you feel the qi.

To finish this Nei Dan, gently guide your attention to the center of the lower Dan Tian, and then continue to move in the Microcosmic Orbit until you feel qi. Finally, complete this cultivation by collecting qi at the center in the lower Dan Tian.

Dai channel Nei Dan part 2

When you feel qi in each of the energy centers in the Dai channel, move to the center of the lower Dan Tian. Then move upward in long spirals, moving up to the crown and above the head in a counter-clockwise flow.

Then reverse the flow, moving clockwise and downward to below the feet. In this process make long spirals, ascending up the channel and then descending down the channel. Repeat this pattern until you feel the qi. Close this mediation by gently moving your attention to the center of the lower Dan Tian and gather qi.

Chapter 24

INNER MEDITATION ON THE CHONG CHANNEL

The Chong channel is also called the "thrusting channel." This channel is the core channel. It is the closest channel to Jing and your *shen*. It can access deep patterns and imprints within a person, and it can be used as a bridge between the interior and exterior, between the prenatal and the postnatal. Clearing and energizing this channel has a profound influence on the three treasures of life. The Chong channel completes the Eight Extraordinary Channels part of this Nei Dan.

The Chong can be viewed in two ways. The first is as one channel. The second way is to view the Chong channel in three sections: the first section is the center, the second section is the right side, and the third is the left side. The Nei Dan process of circulating qi is the same as described for the other channels.

Chong mediation 1

The first Nei Dan method is based on viewing the Chong channel as one channel. Begin by moving your attention to the perineum. As you inhale, guide your attention up to the crown. As you exhale, guide your attention back down to the perineum. Repeat this method of inhaling up and exhaling down 10 times. This comprises one round. Repeat this for up to 9 rounds, or until you feel qi. Feeling qi is the goal. When you feel qi, do this practice a few more rounds until the qi builds. Then, to finish this Nei Dan, bring your attention back to the center in the lower Dan Tian and collect the qi.

Collecting qi in the center of the lower Dan Tian concludes every practice. Your breathing should be done in a relaxed and gentle way. Do not create any stress or rigidity in the body during this practice.

Chong meditation 2

The second method for the Chong channel Nei Dan is to view the channel in three sections (Figure 25.1). The first area is the center of the perineum, and it flows up the center of the body to the center of the brain. The second area is the right side of the perineum, and it flows up the right side of the body to the right side of the brain. The third area is the left side of the perineum, and it flows up the left side of the body.

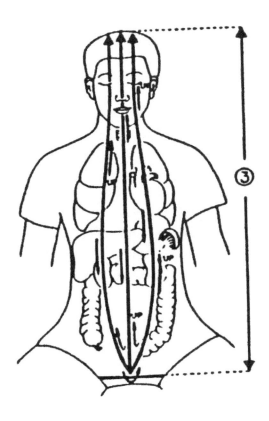

Figure 24.1 The Chong channel

Begin this practice in the center of the perineum. Repeat the same method for each section of the Chong channel. Begin by guiding your attention to the center of the perineum. As you inhale, guide your attention up the center of the body to the center of the brain. As you exhale, guide your attention down the body to the center of the perineum. Then gently move your attention to the right side and repeat the inhalation and exhalation, up and down the right side of the channel. Repeat this process in the center of the perineum, then to the left side of the channel. Then move to the center of the perineum. Repeat this process from the center, right, center, left, and center, 9 times to complete one round. Practice this sequence up to 9 rounds or until you feel the qi.

To finish this part of the Nei Dan, gently guide your attention to the center of the lower Dan Tian. Then move into the Microcosmic Orbit until you feel qi in this orbit pathway. Complete this cultivation by collecting qi in the center of the lower Dan Tian.

⊰⊱

Practice the entire Eight Extraordinary Channels Nei Dan until you feel qi in each of the channels. Follow the exact order given in this and the preceding chapters until you feel qi flowing in all the channels. When you feel qi in all the channels, change the order of practice to the following sequence, which will be the way to practice from now on.

1. Begin in the center in the lower Dan Tian.

2. Du channel.

3. Ren channel.

4. Continue in the orbit until qi is felt.

5. Chong channel.

6. Dai channel.

7. Yin Qiao and Yin Wei channels.

8. Yang Qiao and Yang Wei channels.

9. Circulate qi in the Heavenly Orbit.

10. Close by gathering qi in the center of the lower Dan Tian.

Chapter 25

INNER MEDITATION ON THE MACROCOSMIC ORBIT

The Macrocosmic Orbit adds the legs and arms to the Microcosmic Orbit meditation. This cultivation is added after the Eight Extraordinary Channels Nei Dan has been practiced. It integrates all the channels and the whole body.

After completing the Qiao and Wei channels, gently bring your attention to the center of the lower Dan Tian; collect the qi and follow the following meditation:

1. Form the energy into a qi pearl, the size of a marble or quarter, by spiraling the qi in the lower Dan Tian. With practice you will feel this qi pearl. If you don't feel it, just continue with the practice. You can experiment by making the pearl or energy formation the size of a lemon or orange, it may enhance the feeling and the clearing of the channels. Practice the method that is comfortable.

2. Gently inhale into the center, and then exhale and guide your attention to the perineum.

3. Split your attention/pearl into two parts at the perineum.

4. Exhale down the inside of the legs, to the bottom of the ankle, to the big toe. This pathway down the legs includes the Yin Wei and Yin Qiao channels. You can pause and take a breath or two at the big toe or slightly off the body.

5. When you are ready, inhale up the lateral or external area of the legs along the Yang Qiao and Yang Wei channels, to the shoulder, and to the seventh cervical vertebra at Du 14.

6. Exhale down the lateral areas of the arms to the fingers. Take a breath or two with your attention at the fingertips or a little outside the body.

7. When you are ready, inhale up the interior parts of the arms to the seventh cervical vertebra at Du 14, and continue inhaling up to the crown, which is Du 20.

8. Exhale as you guide your attention down the front of the body, along the Ren channel, to the center of the lower Dan Tian.

9. Inhale into the lower Dan Tian and then exhale, guiding your attention down the Ren channel to the perineum and then down the interior of the legs.

10. With a natural breath inhale up the outer legs to Du 14 (seventh cervical vertebra), and exhale down the exterior areas of the arms to the fingers.

11. Then inhale up the interior aspects of the arms to Du 14, and then up to the crown.

12. Exhale down the center channel/Ren channel to the lower Dan Tian.

Repeat this Macrocosmic Orbit 9 times, or until you feel the qi flowing throughout the Macrocosmic Orbit.

Complete this cultivation by moving into the Microcosmic Orbit for a few circulations, and then collect qi at the center of the lower Dan Tian.

Chapter 26
A Guide to the Inner Landscape Map

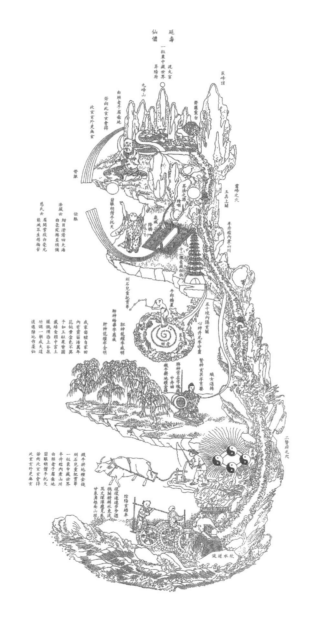

Figure 26.1 The Nei Jing Tu (inner landscape map)

The Nei Jing Tu is a map of the body and its processes. The map illustrates the transformations that occur during Nei Dan or certain types of meditation. The ancient insights can be explained in a variety of ways. I present these processes in a practical, clear way that a wide audience can both understand and apply in their personal cultivation, as well as in clinical practice. Refer to the Nei Jing Tu to have a visual of the areas explained.

1. Gate of Life and Death

This represents the area where our life force can flow downward and out of the body, which drains our remaining life force. Life force can leave in this way via sexual energy and blood. It can leave through the penis, vagina, or anus. Practicing Nei Dan can reverse the flow of the life force, turning it upward to be recycled in the body. This reversal of the flow of life force is the key to health and rejuvenation. It allows qi to be retained and guided through the channels to energize the body. The Microcosmic Orbit Nei Dan assists in directing qi up the back to be recycled in the body.

2. Tail Gate

Life begins in the lower Dan Tian, in the uterus. This area contains Jing, which is the foundation of the body, and it includes Kidney Yin and Kidney Yang. Located at the perineum, there is a boy and a girl. The boy represents Kidney Yang, the testicles, and Jing qi. The girl represents Kidney Yin, the ovaries, and Jing Yin. The boy and girl are turning a waterwheel. The waterwheel represents the process of integrating Yin and Yang (Kidney Yin and Kidney Yang) and pumping it into the Du channel at the coccyx, where it will continue to flow up the body.

In Chinese medicine, the body's Yang (the Gate of Vitality/Ming Men) cooks Jing to create source qi. This source qi is referred to as steam. Source qi is the original qi in the body. It is the foundation of all qi. The quality and quantity of this qi is essential to health and vitality. In Nei Dan, we begin meditating in this area. This helps to make the steaming process more efficient and effective at producing source qi. The boy, the girl, and the waterwheel represent this process of steaming.

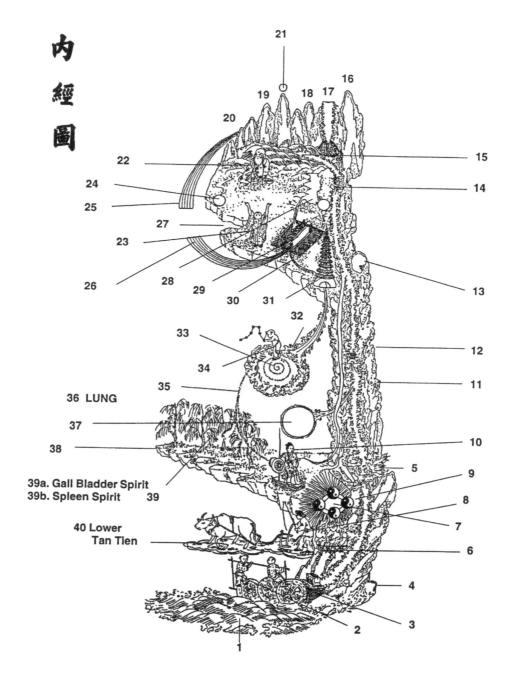

Figure 26.2 The Nei Jing Tu

3–4. Sacral Hiatus Gate

The qi from the Tail Gate flows to the sacral hiatus, Du 2, Yao Shu. This is represented as a rock with eight holes. The rock is the sacrum. The holes in the rock are the eight sacral foramina. The spinal nerves flow into the foramina. An enormous amount of energy flows through this area. These holes are a metaphor for "portals" that receive Earth energies, and then blend them with the Kidney Yin and Yang from the Tail Gate. The Sacral Hiatus Gate includes Jing qi, which includes sexual energy. Jing creates the marrow matrix, which includes marrow and bone. Jing is closely related to bone. Guiding qi to the sacrum infuses the bone with vitality and enhances Jing. The sacrum represents Earth and the lower part of the lower Dan Tian. Moving vital substances to this area is a type of "marrow washing practice." The sacrum acts as a pump that moves qi up the spine. This area has a strong influence on Jing, bone, source qi, fertility, and the genitals.

5. Gate of Destiny

The qi from the Sacral Hiatus Gate moves to the Kidneys and Ming Men, Du 4. The Ming Men is the Gate of Vitality and the Fire of the body. This Fire (Yang) ignites the process of Yang cooking Yin. The Fire cooks Jing, which creates source qi. This gate has a strong influence on the Kidneys, both Yang and Yin. "Ming" means destiny. In a Nei Dan context, destiny means the quality of our life force. Nei Dan influences the quality of our life. Destiny includes hereditary and ancestral influences. Cultivating this gate and cultivating the entire lower Dan Tian can release ancestral influences. We can transform and move beyond them. By refining the qi, the energetics and influences inside Jing are transformed to a neutral state. This is the qi stage in the Jing-qi-*shen* process.

6. The Cauldron

This is the lower Dan Tian cauldron. This is where the Ming Men cooks Jing, creating source qi. This area also activates sexual qi (which comes from Jing). In Nei Dan, we bring internal energies together. This cauldron serves to conserve, refine, and move them. This cauldron is where we mix and blend our life force to rejuvenate our body. This refined qi becomes the basis of our life, our awareness, and our consciousness.

7. Yin–Yang and Tai Chi

The four Yin–Yang/Tai Chi symbols represent the moving force inside our body. This natural force assists in the transformation of Jing to qi to *shen*. This force activates the Ming Men, the Gate of Vitality. Ming Men cooks Jing, creating steam or source qi. In Nei Dan terminology, we call this creation of source qi "steaming."

8. Buffalo Plows the Land and Plants the Golden Elixir

This gate is opposite the navel area, at the back. It is a bridge from the Kidneys, Jing, sexual qi, source qi, the Spleen/Stomach center, and the *yi*. It includes the relationship between prenatal and postnatal. When sexual qi and source qi move into the Du channel and flow up the spine, source qi also moves to the Earth center/the Spleen, and Stomach. Earth is the transforming element. In Nei Dan, the function of Earth is to transform Jing into qi. This is the first stage in the Nei Dan process of Jing-qi-*shen*. In Chinese medicine, this center creates Gu qi. Gu qi then rises up to the Lungs and Heart. This rising of qi is essential to create qi and blood in the body. The Earth center houses the *yi*. The *yi* is our intellectual capacity. It is our thinking and thoughts. The *yi* filters all experiences of life. It organizes and digests life experiences. Understanding this process enables us to realize how we process life experiences. The Nei Dan process can assist in changing how we process these experiences. Awareness of the process can also help in releasing ourselves from attachments to old patterns and imprints from early life and from current stresses and intensities. Nei Dan refines our life force, the *yi*, and our filtering process. This refined life force can connect to our Yuan Shen. This process allows patterns, imprints, and stresses to become conscious, allowing them to be transformed. More importantly, we have the opportunity to see them as patterns, imprints, and stresses, rather than part of our essential nature. The Earth center is the link from the lower Dan Tian to the upper Dan Tian. If stagnations, blockages, or other aspects of conditioning are not transformed, they will go to the Heart center. This will subsequently influence our Heart *shen*.

9. The True Dan Tian

This is the location of the Elixir Field. It is the area above the cauldron at the four Tai Chi symbols; it is closer to the spine. This area is where the body's heat creates steam. Qi is represented pictorially as the steam rising from Fire cooking rice. This image of steam is an essential aspect of Nei Dan.

10. Weaving Maiden Spins at her Loom

This area is the right Kidney, which is Yin and Water. Above the maiden is the cowherder, which represents Yang at the Heart level. The weaving maiden gathers Yin from the body, the stars, the planets, and the cosmos. This Yin is then stored in the lower Dan Tian. One's intention, breath, and body (for example, the eyes) are used to gather and store vital substances in the lower Dan Tian. This gate is where the Yin of the Kidneys and the Yang of the Heart unite. This unification is the mingling of *shen* and Jing, which nourishes the transformation of Jing-qi-*shen*.

11. The Kidney Zhi Spirit

This area reflects the Kidneys' ability to store prenatal energies, which then transport those energies to support our spiritual development. The Kidneys contain the *zhi* and willpower. Your willpower helps you live the life you desire.

12. Gate to the One

This area is located opposite the Heart. It is an area where qi can be drawn into the Heart and the Heart center.

13. The Big Hammer

This is Da Zhui, the Big Hammer, Du 14. It is at the seventh vertebra. It is where all the Yang channels intersect. Da Zhui connects the lower center to the upper center, and then connects the trunk to the arms. This area needs to be clear and free flowing, to let qi circulate to the upper Dan Tian and the arms.

14. Cave of the Spirit Peak

This area is Yao Men, Mute's Gate, Du 15. There is an internal pathway that flows from this point to the brain. It has a strong influence on Jing-Shen, the brain. This area guides qi to the upper Dan Tian and assists in the transformation of Jing-qi-*shen*. This center assists us in self-expression.

15. Sea of Marrow

The whole head is a mountain with nine caves. The Sea of Marrow surrounds the crown of the head. It includes areas behind, in front of, and to the sides of the crown. This area is where heavenly energies flow into our body. An alchemical image includes nine caves. We practice Nei Dan in these caves and centers.

16. Top of the Great Peak

This area contains the pineal gland, which is an "internal compass" in Nei Dan. This inner compass connects to the North Star, and the center of the sky/celestial. This area connects to heavenly energy. We can make this connection by tucking our chin inward and tilting our head upward.

17. High Place of Many Veils

The High Place of the Many Veils is where the spirit and soul can either exit or enter. It is between the Great Peak and the Muddy Pill.

18. Muddy Pill

Muddy Pill is located at Bai Hui, Hundred Meetings, Du 20. When this area is open, it feels like soft mud. It includes the hypothalamus gland. It is a conduit to draw qi inward, as well as project qi outward. It connects to the Big Dipper.

19. House of Rising Yang

This is the third eye (Yin Tang). Yin Tang receives energies from the sun and the moon. It is the center of psychic powers, and it is a conduit to the exterior.

20. Nine Sacred Peaks

This location is near the mid-eyebrow. The area includes the pituitary gland; it receives energies to travel in the earthly planes.

21. Immortal Realm

This is the area in front of the crown. The Immortal Realm can draw heavenly energies into the body.

22. Lao Zi

Lao Zi is the Old Man. He is the founder of philosophical Taoism. He is located in the celestial (head) and his long, white beard flows to the Earth. Lao Zi is a living embodiment of the unity of Heaven and Earth. As he lives in the Way (The Tao), he becomes the Way.

23. Heaven and Earth Destiny

This is Damo extending his hands up to connect to the heavenly energy. Damo and Lao Zi are the founders of philosophical Taoism and Chan Buddhism (Chinese Buddhism). Both represent the integration of our heavenly and earthly destination.

24. Sun and Moon Within

The two circles above Damo are the sun and the moon. They are Yang and Yin. The sun and the moon are also the left and right eyes. By moving the eyes in Nei Dan, we move the Yang and Yin energies in the body. The eye movement integrates and mingles Yang and Yin, which creates harmony. In Nei Dan, the eyes are used to look inside the body. This "looking" guides qi. When we spiral at various areas of the body, the eyes likewise spiral, which enhances the effects of circulating, gathering, and collecting.

25 and 26. Du and Ren channels

The Du and Ren channels are the major Yin and Yang channels. They are represented here as thick channels lying above, below, and in front of Lao Zi. These two channels comprise the Microcosmic Orbit (small Heavenly Orbit).

27. The Drawbridge

This is the tongue. It is sometimes called the "Pool of Water." When the tongue touches the palate, it connects the Ren and Du channels. This allows energies to flow through the Microcosmic Orbit and the three Dan Tian. This bridge generates fluids, which are the result of Nei Dan. The fluids change from saliva, to nectar, and then to elixir. With practice, the body generates and accumulates increased levels of qi. This influences the organs, glands, and our body fluids. As we cultivate our life force, our qi and body fluids change.

28. Dew Pond

This area is located behind the soft palate and connects to the pituitary gland.

29. Mouth Pool

This is Yin Jiao, Gum Intersection, Du 28. It is the area where the elixir flows from the Dew Pond. Cosmic energy enters here during breathing.

30. Heavenly Pool

This is the area where the tongue connects to the palate. This area brings saliva to the palate.

31. The Pagoda

This is Tian Tu, Heaven's Chimney, Ren 22. It is located in the space at the top of the sternum. The qi flowing in the heavenly orbit flows down the throat through this area to nourish the Heart.

32. Flaming Balls of Fire

This area is around the "Cowherder Boy Connects to the Stars" (see 34 below). It represents the Nei Dan cultivation at the Heart center. This Nei Dan contains the Fire and passion of our quest for self-realization.

33. Spiral of Rice Grains

The rice grain is a metaphor for the microcosm. All of life is inside each person. Learning to focus our life with Nei Dan enables us to understand both Heaven and Earth. The ways of Earth are called nature. The ways of Heaven are called destiny. The way of the Tao is the cultivation and integration of both Heaven and Earth, which allows one to enjoy the fruits of all aspects of life.

34. Cowherder Boy Connects to the Stars

This area reflects the connection of the Heart *shen*, love, and compassion. The stars reflect our connection to the Big Dipper and the heavenly realm. Aligning to the Big Dipper during the year enables us to connect to and gather heavenly energies, to support our Nei Dan practice.

35. Milky Way

This is a bridge connecting the Heart and the Kidneys, connecting the Yang and Yin, and connecting the Water and Fire. The Heart and the

Kidneys are Shao Yin. This connection reflects Jing seeking *shen*, and it reflects the will for self-realization. The Milky Way merges the Kidney *zhi* and the Heart *shen*.

36. Lung Spirit

The Lung Spirit represents the value of releasing. When the Lungs inhale, they fill with cosmic qi; when they exhale, they empty. Emptying is essential to health, vitality, and self-realization. Being empty allows each breath, and each moment, to be new and rejuvenating.

37. Solar Plexus

The Solar Plexus is the middle Dan Tian. It includes the Spleen, Stomach, Liver, Gallbladder, and the *hun* and the *yi*.

38. Outer Ring of the Forest

This area is the edge of the rib cage. It is where the diaphragm is housed.

39. Liver Spirit

The trees are the Wood element, and they correspond to the Liver. The Liver stores and transports qi and blood. Its function includes creating the smooth flow of qi and blood. It also supports the smooth flow of emotions. The Kidneys are the Water element. They nourish Wood and the Liver, which in turn nourishes the Heart: this is Wood nourishing Fire. The Liver is the general, and a good general has a good plan. Nei Dan cultivation reveals a plan, and a direction in life.

39a. Gallbladder Spirit

This area is in the middle of the Liver. The Liver and the Gallbladder open to the eyes. The outer eyes are eyesight; the inner eyes are spiritual clarity. The Gallbladder is essential in obtaining clarity. Nei Dan cultivates our ability to be clear and decisive.

39b. Spleen Spirit

This location is at the Spleen area. It relates to the *yi* and the transformation process. Nei Dan transforms and refines. As the *yi* becomes refined with Nei Dan practice, we are able to be a living expression of the Way/the Tao.

40. Lower Dan Tian

This area represents the alchemy of the lower Sea of Qi. "The Cauldron," "Yin–Yang and Tai Chi," and "Buffalo Plows the Land and Plants the Golden Elixir" represent the Nei Dan process.

❊

The processes in the Nei Jing Tu and our body continue throughout our lifetime. The flow of seas, rivers, streams, springs, and wells is the exterior image of the interior flows of vital substances: Jing, qi, blood, and body fluids. Proper flows of Water are essential to life and a bountiful harvest. Optimal circulation of the vital substances is a key to health and vitality. The Eight Extraordinary Channels Nei Dan is a powerful way to assist in creating effective circulation of vital substances. This healthy flow clears the rough, allowing you to see and experience the diamond shining inside. This Nei Dan assists in fulfilling our life quest, and achieving self-realization.

AFTERWORD

I was first introduced to the Eight Extraordinary Channels while studying Taoist meditation. These channels are also called "the eight psychic channels." They are the links between Jing and *shen*. I was fortunate to learn about these channels from that viewpoint; it gave me a very wide view of their functions. Most importantly, I was able to feel them. I have taught workshops and retreats on this inner meditation (Nei Dan). These practices have had a profound influence on the participants, as well as myself. It is my favorite meditation to practice and teach.

The Eight Extraordinary Channels are an essential aspect of Chinese medicine and Nei Dan. I wrote this book for three main reasons. The first is to present a practical guide to help practitioners use the Eight Extraordinary Channels in clinical practice. The second is to provide information to people interested in learning more about healing, qi gong, meditation, and Nei Dan (inner meditation). And the third reason is to create a bridge between the practice of Chinese medicine, with a focus on the psycho-emotional and spiritual aspects of our life, and Nei Dan inner meditation. Understanding this bridge allows the practitioner of Chinese medicine to assist in the life path of each patient. It also provides a person with a deeper insight to the inner workings of their cultivation practices.

I hope this book assists you in your clinical practice, meditation, and spiritual path. Feel free to contact me via my website www.healingqi.com with questions and feedback on this book.

With best wishes,
David Twicken

BIBLIOGRAPHY

Bertschinger, R. (2011) *The Secret of Everlasting Life: The First Translation of the Ancient Chinese Text of Immorality*. London: Singing Dragon.

Chace, C. and Shima, M. (2010) *An Exposition on the Eight Extraordinary Vessels: Acupuncture, Alchemy, and Herbal Medicine*. Seattle, WA: Eastland Press.

Chia, M. (1983) *Awaken Healing Energy through the Tao*. Santa Fe, NM: Aurora Press.

Chia, M. (1995) *Inner Alchemy of the Tao*. Chiang Mai, Thailand: Healing Tao Co. Ltd.

Chia, M. (2009) *Fusion of the Eight Psychic Channels: Opening and Sealing the Energy Body*. Rochester, VT: Destiny Books.

Ellis, A., Wiseman, N. and Boss, K. (1989) *Grasping the Wind: An Exploration into the Meaning of Chinese Acupuncture Point Names*. Brookline, MA: Paradigm Publications.

Harper, D. (2007) *Early Chinese Medical Literature: The Mawangdui Medical Manuscripts*. London: Kegan Paul International.

Jacob, J. (1996) *The Acupuncturist's Clinical Handbook*. Integrative Wellness.

Johnson, J.A. (2000) *Chinese Medical Qi Gong Therapy*. Pacific Grove, CA: International Institute of Medical Qi Gong.

Komjathy, L. (2008) "Mapping the Daoist Body (1): The *Neijing tu* in History." *Journal of Daoist Studies 1*, 67–92.

Komjathy, L. (2009) "Mapping the Daoist Body (2): The Text of the *Neijing tu*." *Journal of Daoist Studies 2*, 64–108.

Larre, C., Rochat de la Vallee, E. and Hill, S. (1997) *The Eight Extraordinary Meridians*. Monkey Press.

Luk, C. and Yu, K.Y. (1999) *Taoist Yoga: Alchemy and Immortality*. San Francisco, CA: Red Wheel/Weiser.

Maciocia, G. (2006) *The Channels of Acupuncture: Clinical Use of the Secondary Channels and the Eight Extraordinary Vessels*. Oxford: Churchill Livingstone.

Matsumoto, K. and Birch, S. (1986) *Eight Extraordinary Channels*. Brookline, MA: Paradigm Publications.

Ni, Y. (1996) *Navigating the Channels of Traditional Chinese Medicine.* San Diego, CA: Complementary Medicine Press.

Schipper, K. (1994) *The Taoist Body.* Berkeley, CA: University of California Press.

Twicken, D. (2002) *Treasures of Tao.* Bloomington, IN: iUniverse.

Twicken, D. (2011) *I Ching Acupuncture: The Balance Method. Clinical Applications of the Ba Gua and I Ching.* London: Jessica Kingsley Publishers.

Veith, I. (1966) *The Yellow Emperor's Classic of Internal Medicine.* Berkeley, CA: University of California Press.

Wang, S.-H and Yang, S. (1997) *The Pulse Classic: A Translation of the Mai Jing.* Boulder, CO: Blue Poppy Press.

Wu, J. (2002) *Ling Shu or The Spiritual Pivot.* Hawaii: University of Hawaii Press.

Wu, N. and Wu, A. (2002) *Yellow Emperor's Canon of Internal Medicine.* Beijing, China: China Science Technology Press.

Yang, C. (2004) *A Systematic Classic of Acupuncture and Moxibustion.* Boulder, CO: Blue Poppy Press.

INDEX